Mini H

Lorraine Ellis

chipmunkapublishing
the mental health publisher

Published by
Chipmunkapublishing
PO Box 6872
Brentwood
Essex CM13 1ZT
United Kingdom

http://www.chipmunkapublishing.com

Chipmunkapublishing gratefully acknowledge the support of Arts Council England.

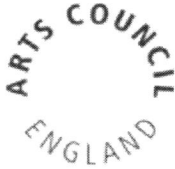

Some of the names in this autobiography have been changed.

Lorraine Ellis

Acknowledgements

I would like to thank my family for their encouragement and support.
And a big thanks to my daughter Lucy Ellis for the drawing on the front cover.

Lorraine Ellis

Author Biography

Lorraine Ellis, mother of three, was born in Hull in 1957.

At the age of fifteen Lorraine had a breakdown in her mental health and was admitted to a psychiatric hospital where she was diagnosed as to be suffering from a schizophrenic attack. She recovered after six months and was well for many years. She married and had a young family. However in her late twenties mental illness reared its ugly head. And she was re -diagnosed with manic depression. Over the next seventeen years Lorraine suffered many attacks and had frequent admissions to hospital. During her attacks she became delusional and heard voices in her head.

She describes them as terrible times where there was no escape.

In order to elude the voices Lorraine was driven to desperate measures which led to a three month stay in a general hospital and wheelchair bound for many months.

During her recovery Lorraine spent most of her time writing and working on her novel Pease Pudding Hot which she finished shortly after moving to a small east Yorkshire village with her husband of thirty three years. She is now maintained on tablets which she will take for the rest of her life but fortunately has been reasonably well for the last seven years, Recently Lorraine has since completed two short autobiographies entitled Mini Hen legs and Ladybird Ladybird fly away home. Mini hen legs concentrates on childhood to adolescence . Her second biography Ladybird Ladybird fly away home, focuses on Lorraine's adulthood and family life. She hopes her work will give people an insight in how it feels to become mentally unwell and help to eradicate the stigma that is attached to this illness. Lorraine also hopes to help other suffers feel that are not so alone.

Lorraine Ellis

1962
Chapter 1

It is still dark; I can hear Mammy's light footsteps on the stairs. Although I'm awake I close my eyes tightly, even put my thumb into my mouth so that she will think I'm still sleeping. I only suck my thumb at bedtimes because my Dad says that big girls don't do that. And yes, I am a big girl now, for today I'm starting school. I had laid awake for most of last night, I still wasn't asleep when the big clock struck eleven; but now its morning all I want to do is sleep.
Mammy stands by my bed. I can hear her breathing.
'Come on Mini hen legs, it's time you were getting up.'
'I've got a tummy ache,' I mutter, wanting to slip back into the cosy warmth of my bed.'
Mammy takes no notice so hesitantly I climb out of my bed.

Having managed to swallow two spoonfuls of porridge, I wash and brush my teeth. When Mammy has checked that my neck is clean I put on my liberty bodice. Mammy helps to fasten the row of rubber buttons at the front. 'This will keep your back warm,' she says. I don't like the liberty bodice. It feels hard and uncomfortable against my skin, and by the time Mammy has finished fastening the thing I really do have a tummy ache.

My new kilt has a large silver safety pin at the side of it. We bought it last Monday from town, along with the starchy white blouses which I'm to wear beneath the grey cardigan that Aunty Audrey has knitted me.
We called in at Aunty Audrey's on the way home from town and I played with little Audrey and Susan who are my cousins. I have a lot of cousins; some of them live down our street. Sometimes we go and see my Uncle Bill and Auntie Peggy and my cousins Diane, Carole and John. My cousin Diane has left school now and she says that when she gets married I can be her bridesmaid.

The cardigan is soft but it doesn't fit very well and hangs down almost to my knees. The sleeves are also very long, and the cuffs have to be turned over two and a half times.

'She'll soon grow into it' Aunty Audrey had clucked when Mammy tried it on me.

'Yes, it's a good fit our Audrey,' agreed Mammy, 'it will last her longer.'

I'd sulked and pouted all the way home from Aunt Audrey's and our shopping trip because I didn't like the grey cardigan and I wanted Mammy to buy me the turquoise dress with the pretty silky sash, and a pair of the fancy ankle socks. But Mammy had said that those clothes weren't suitable for school. So we arrived home with the misshapen cardigan and sensible school clothes; three pairs of long navy socks and a pair of equally sensible T bar shoes, dull brown with sharp edged buckles. I wished my cousin Diane would hurry and get married, then I would wear a lovely silky bridesmaid dress and fancy white shoes.

*****

Now I'm all dressed in my new clothes Mammy takes her hairbrush and sits me on her knee.

My hair hangs down in thin little wisps around my face. Mammy sweeps it upwards and then taking the grips from out of her mouth. She fastens it up with a large red ribbon.

'You look like an Easter egg,' laughs my Dad.

'Don't tease her,' said Mammy giving him a quick swipe around his lug. 'She looks beautiful, don't you?' she smiles. 'You look beautiful and so grown up too, go and have a peep in the mirror.'

Mammy turns around and dabs her eyes and Dad lifts me up so that I can see myself in the large mirror above our mantelpiece.

I stare in the mirror. I look so different with my hair scraped back off my face and now I don't have a fringe the large freckles on my forehead are very noticeable. As I look into the mirror I can see Grahame standing by the sideboard sniggering and I feel anything but beautiful.

My bottom lip wobbles as I put on my coat; Mammy put my plimsoll bag on my shoulder and gives me a silver sixpence and a threepenny bit.

'That's your dinner money,' she said, 'You must give that to Miss Barrat.'

I can feel hot tears pricking my eyes and I swallow back the lump in my throat as I realise that there will be no more 'Tales From the

River Bank,' 'Andy Pandy', or 'Woodentops', because I'm a big girl now and big girls go to school and don't watch baby programmes.

'Come on love,' says Mammy, taking my hand.
We reach the end of our terrace then head towards the school at the top of our street, where I will soon begin my very first day. Grahame runs on in front me with the gangling giggling gang of older boys and girls. He doesn't want to be seen walking with Mammy, because he's been going to school all by himself for a long time now.
Mammy waves goodbye to me as she walks away from the school gates. I see her turn around, just the once. I watch her as she reaches the corner shop and then she disappears inside. I then realise that I haven't had anything off the penny tray. I like going into Mrs Bailoid's shop; Mammy takes me there every day. She has a large silver tray which she brings out from beneath the counter. It has lots of different goodies on it all costing one penny and Mammy always lets me choose one. It's very noisy in the playground. I put my hands over my ears and I have a funny feeling in my tummy. I want to run back out of the large iron gates, chase down the street and dash into Mrs Bailoid's, but that's not just because I want to choose something from the penny tray.

'Anybody in the way gets a big kick!' A group of big boys are marching towards me, their arms linked. I walk backwards until my back rests on the wall and edge towards the end of the playground, away from their long legs and dirty boots.
Suddenly a high pitched whistle fills my ears and the boys stop dead in their tracks, and now there's a silence in the grey playground.
'Would the new boys and girls line up outside the blue door!' shouts a lady with a silver whistle dangling from her neck on a piece of string. I stay where I am against the cold wall and watch as kids form perfect straight lines and make their way into their classrooms.
Very soon apart from the lady with the dangling whistle I am the only one left in the playground.
'Are you one of the little 'uns,' I shrug my shoulders because Dad did say that I'm a big girl now.

'Is this your first day?'
'Oh yes, yes it is.'

'Yes Miss Wood,' said the teacher.
'Y e s Miss W w oo d,' I reply.
'What's your name?' asks Miss Wood.
'Min..,' I stutter.
Miss Wood frowns. 'Speak up child,' she says.
' Mi.. I mean Lorraine,' I quickly add, remembering to tell her my real name and not my nickname, the name I'm more familiar with.
'And your surname?'
I shift from foot to foot.
'Your second name child, what's your second name.'
'Oh, that's Tranmer,' I reply, 'and my full name is Lorraine Florence Tranmer.'
Miss Wood smiles. 'Mm Lorraine Florence, why you have the name of two beautiful cities child.'

Miss wood has brought me to my classroom. I'm sitting next to a girl called Sally Clarke.
Sally Clarke never gave the teacher any dinner money because she said that she was going home for her dinner. My teacher's name is Mrs Barret. She has a wide mouth that smiles a lot and her eyes dance and twinkle and I think I like her more than Miss Wood.
We are in the school hall and I have just got changed into my plimsolls. Sally helped me unbutton the liberty bodice and I have tucked my vest in my navy blue knickers. I don't like the navy blue knickers; they look like old coal bags.
'Children, I want you all to curl up in a tight little ball, then slowly uncurl.'
The teacher plays some music and we all uncurl and slowly stand up.
'Wave your arms children like trees, trees blowing in the wind.'
I think about the trees in the park and sway my arms to the music.
We're getting dressed now. I put my liberty bodice back on but I can't fasten the buttons and Sally is in the toilet so I leave them open and just slip my blouse over the top. I don't think I have fastened my skirt properly either, it feels so loose and strange and I have trouble keeping it up as I climb down the stairs towards my classroom.
Sally's gone home for her dinner, some of the others have as well. The rest of us along with Miss wood, and the two dinner ladies Mrs Jenkins and Mrs Winterson form a line and leave the iron gate. We stand at the side of the road just opposite Kings Hall, the place

where I go to Sunday School.

Miss Wood blows her whistle. 'At the kerb halt. Look right, look left. When all is clear...'

Miss Wood tells us all to turn to see if we can see any traffic, then we all cross the road, but Miss Wood knew that there were no cars coming anyway.

'Do not run!' she shouts at a ginger haired boy near the front of the line.

We enter Kings Hall and walk up the corridor, passing the small room where the Sunday school class is held. The main hall looks so different now with the rows of tables and chairs. The last time I was in this large room was when we had the Sunday school party. I felt so excited and happy that day, but I don't feel very happy now, or excited.

'For what we are about to receive may the lord make us truly grateful,' chants Miss Wood. We all say 'amen'. I open my eyes and glance down quickly noticing that the big silver pin is missing off my new kilt and I hope that Mammy isn't going to be cross.

A big boy and girl sit opposite each other at the front of our table. They are the servers and they ladle out the mashed potatoes and vegetables from large oblong shaped silver containers, along with slices of meat from a wide silver dish.

'Small or large?' asks the server.

I shrug my shoulders and stare at the plastic checked table-cloth so the girl server gets on with serving me my dinner.

'Oh no, it's liver and onions,' says a girl sitting by my side.

The gravy jug is passed around. I'm the last to get it and when it comes to my turn there is hardly any gravy left, not even enough to cover the two pale grey mounds of mashed potato. We all have a plastic cup which we fill with water from the jug in the middle of the table. There are bits of turnip and potato floating on the top, but I'm very thirsty so I fill my cup up and sip some. It's luke warm and tastes a bit like plastic. The big girl helps me to cut my meat. It tastes nasty so I take another drink of the water to wash it down my throat, the plastic flavour tasting better then the meat. I slip a couple of tiny forkfuls of turnip into my mouth. It doesn't taste like turnip, not the turnip Mammy makes; all I can taste is pepper. I don't eat any more and just spread the mounds of potato around my plate until it's all flat. My tummy is rumbling, I'm hungry but I still don't eat much of the dinner.

It's rice pudding for sweet, I'm glad, I like rice pudding, and this looks nice and creamy, it's got a big dollop of jam in the middle. My mouth is watering and the rumbling and grumbling in my tummy is getting louder.

I'm just going to dip my spoon into my rice pudding when I see Sally Clarke and a tall lady enter the hall. The lady is holding Sally's hand as she stands talking to Mrs Winterson, the dinner lady. They're looking my way and pointing. I put my spoon down as they stop at our table.

'Will you just stand up for a moment Please?' asks Mrs Winterson nodding her head in my direction. I get up quickly, scraping the legs of my chair until it clatters back on to the stone floor of the hall. Everyone has stopped talking and all the kids in the hall are staring at me.

The tall lady looks at me from head to toe, her eyes resting on my middle. 'Yes, that's the one,' she says to Mrs Winterson.

'Come here,' says Mrs Winterson.

I stand at the front of the table whilst Mrs Winterson takes my skirt off and the tall lady takes off Sally's skirt.

'I don't know, we have got into a muddle this morning.' The tall lady is smiling now.

Our skirts are quickly swapped, I then realise that I must have put Sally Clarke's skirt on by mistake.

Everyone on my table is laughing. I feel my face burning. I bite my bottom lip because I feel ashamed and my rice pudding has gone cold, and now has a horrible thick skin on the top of it.

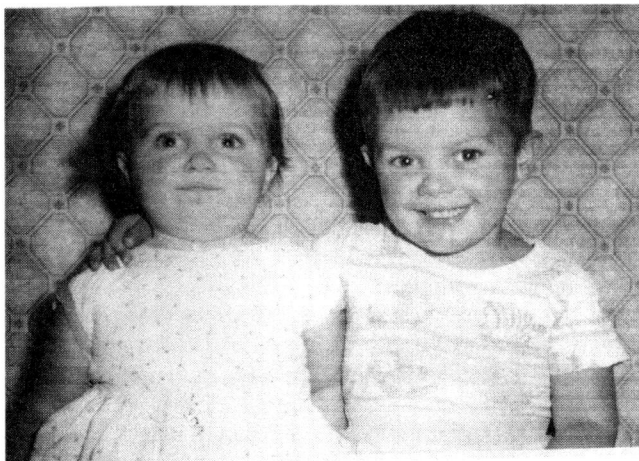

Grahame and Lorraine Tranmer 1960

Chapter 2

'There's one!' shouts Mammy pulling up strands of my hair.
'There's another, oh My God she's infested with 'em.'
The steel comb scrapes my scalp making it tingle and raw.
'Got the bugger,' Mammy sighs disgustedly. 'That's four I've got so far but they move that fast it will take me forever to catch them all.'
'What are you getting Mammy?' I ask bewildered, 'What are you getting out of my hair?'
Mammy ignores me, her face grim with concentration. She continues to pull up strands of my wispy hair.
'Ouch!'
'Keep still love,, damn, I nearly had that bugger.'
'Mammy!' I say in surprise, 'That was a naughty word.'
'Be quiet Lorraine that's a good lass, and try to keep still.'
'But what are you getting Mammy? What are you getting out of my hair?'
'You've got dicks, blooming lodgers!' yells Mammy.
'Dicks?' what are di...'
'Little creatures, insects that sometimes live in people's hair.'
Mammy then begins to scrape the comb through my hair again.
Something small drops on to the brown paper that is spread out in front of me on the mat.
'There's one, look!' cries Mammy, who then cracks the offending creature between two finger nails.
'Mammy Mammy! You shouldn't have done that, Mrs Harris at my Sunday school, well she says that it's wicked to kill God's creatures.'
Ignoring me Mammy turns to my Auntie Maud who is sitting on our settee.
'Two weeks, I tell yer, two weeks at that blooming school and she's come home lousy.'
'Did you get the Derback lass?' says Auntie Maud. 'That should see 'em   off.'
Mammy puts a towel around my shoulders and the smelly slimy stuff is slapped on top of my head.
'Best leave it on a while,' says Auntie Maud. 'That should do the trick, there's no need to half scalp the poor little bugger.' Auntie Maud laughs and gives me a Cadbury's flake.

'You smell like mucky Mary,' says Grahame as he comes into the room.

'Mucky Mary?' says Mammy, 'Who's Mucky Mary?'

'Oh mucky Mary, she's in our class, she's always picking and scratching her head, she never gets washed and she's always getting sent to The White Hunter.'

'Poor little bugger,' says Auntie Maud.

'White Hunter comes round every other Thursday,' went on Grahame, 'so she should be coming the day after tomorrow.'

Mammy frowns,' Grahame who on earth is this White Hunter?'

'Oh, the dick nurse, she wears a white coat and she hunts in your hair for dicks.'

'I see,' says Mammy.

'But Mucky Mary, well Jon Spencer says that she's got fleas as well, an' she's got big scabs in her head an'....'

'Grahame!' shouts Mammy, 'That's not very nice.'

'Well, she has.' Grahame's face is turning a little pink.

'Yes, but you mustn't tease the poor little lass, that's mean.' says Auntie Maud.

'I don't,' says Grahame, 'I'm just telling you what Jon Spencer told me, an' I only call her Mucky Mary when she's not listening.'

'You shouldn't ever call her names like that,' says Mammy

'Well she is mu...'

'Get to bed Grahame.'

'Bu...'

'When you get to your room sit and think how you would like it if you were teased like that.'

Grahame slams the door behind him and Mammy throw her arms in the air. 'That's it!' she says, 'She's not going back to that school until she's clean.'

'Good idea,' says Auntie Maud. 'Bairns can be so cruel.'

Mammy says that I can stay in bed, I can hear Grahame getting ready for school.

He lay by my side last night and rubbed his head into mine for ages. But I heard Mammy checking his head earlier and he hasn't caught the dicks; so he has to go to school. He says it's 'not fair', but I'm glad.

Chapter 3

I'm so happy and excited because Uncle Ralph is coming tomorrow to take me and Grahame to the big park, the one that's got the paddling pool and the big splash boat.

I like my Uncle Ralph. He isn't my real uncle, he's my Dad's friend. Mammy says that we must call him Uncle Ralph and not just Ralph as that's polite. She says that 'It isn't nice for kids to call grown ups by their first name.'

I look out of the window watching for Uncle Ralph. At last I see him

'He's here!' I squeal as I run out of the door. Uncle Ralph is walking up our street.

'Hello cherub,' he says as I reach him.

I walk back into the house chattering excitedly to Uncle Ralph. 'Are we going on the splash boat? Will you push me as high as the sky on the swings? Can we feed the ducks? Can I go in the paddling pool?'

'No, ' interrupts Mammy, 'You must keep away from the paddling pool, it's a bit dirty.'

'Never mind,' said Uncle Ralph seeing my look of disappointment, 'there are plenty more nice things we can do.'

I watch Mammy as she butters the bread and spreads it with potted meat, which she cuts it up into tiny sandwiches and then wraps them in greaseproof paper and puts them in a bag along with crisps, biscuits and a big bottle of lemonade.

'Off you go then,' she smiles, kissing me goodbye. 'Be good.'

She passes Uncle Ralph the bag containing our picnic

'I'll be as good as gold, I promise,' I say as we leave the house.

'So will I Mam,' says Grahame.

It's a very warm day and the park is full of laughing boys and girls.

'Push me higher, I want to swing right over the bar!'

I watch in wonder as Uncle Ralph pushes Grahame in the swing faster and faster. I'm happy to swing gently to and fro. I'm too scared to go as high as Grahame.

The sun is getting hot and the paddling pool glistens temptingly.

'Would you like to go for a little paddle?' asks Uncle Ralph.

I nod my head 'I would love to,' I say jumping up and down.

I then remember what Mammy had said.

'It's all right, go and have a little splash, I won't tell your Mammy,' says Uncle Ralph.

I run to the pool. The water is sparkling blue.

I paddle round the edge of the pool but it is a bit dirty as someone has thrown in their empty fish and chip paper. Cigarette ends float on top of the water.

Suddenly I feel someone push me from behind and I fall down into the pool.

I sit in the water crying as my best dress is all wet through and I know Mammy will be very cross with me. Uncle Ralph has his trousers rolled up and he has waded into the pool. He helps me to stand up.

'Who pushed you?' said Grahame.

'I didn't see,' I cry, 'someone came from behind me.'

'Never mind,' said Uncle Ralph. 'I'll take you back to my flat and you can get your clothes dried, then your Mammy won't ever know that you have been in the pool when you know you shouldn't have been.'

We got a taxi back to Uncle Ralph's flat. I'm soaking wet through.

Uncle Ralph keeps laughing at me and shaking his head. 'Never mind,' he says, 'you'll soon be nice and dry.

Very soon we arrive at Uncle Ralph's. His flat is up some stairs above a fish and chip shop. It smells horrible and makes me feel sick.

'Grahame will you go to shop and get me a pint of milk?' asks Uncle Ralph.

He gives Grahame some money and tells him to go to the shop at the top of Charles Street as he says that the milk in the corner shop tastes funny. He also gives Grahame four empty lemonade bottles to take back to a shop in the next street.

'Right, let's get you all nice and dry,' says Uncle Ralph as Grahame leaves the flat.

He begins to take off my wet clothes.

'I can undress myself,' I say, 'I'm a big girl now.'

But Uncle Ralph didn't seem to hear me and unbuttons my wet dress and pulls it over my head. He then takes off the rest of my clothes. I look around the room.

My best dress is lying crumpled and dirty on the grey canvas which lines the floor.

I watch as Uncle Ralph gets up and bolts the door.

Uncle Ralph walks towards me he pulls me in his arms and holds me really tight. It's not like a cuddle Mammy or Dad gives me. It feels horrible and I can hardly breathe.

Suddenly he lets me go. 'Close your eyes!' he shouts, not sounding at all like Uncle Ralph, 'Close your eyes now.'

Trying not to cry I close my eyes.

Uncle Ralph holds me again. I can smell the sweat on his body mingling with the smell coming from the fish and chip shop. I want to be sick..

I open my eyes Uncle Ralph has pulled his trousers down. Maybe he has to get dry. Maybe that's why he keeps cuddling me so tightly. 'Don't look down!' he shouts. 'Close your eyes.'

I look down and I can see his 'thing'.

Someone is knocking at the door. Uncle Ralph lets go of me, pulls up his trousers and puts his finger to his lip. 'Hush now,' he says, 'keep quiet.' The knocking is getting louder and louder.

Suddenly I hear my brother's voice, 'Uncle Ralph, It's me!'

Uncle Ralph opens the door.

'The shop down Charles Street is closed and the other shop wouldn't take the bottles back,' I hear Grahame say.

'Well then try the shop further up the street.' Uncle Ralph closes the door in my brother's face.

'Can you keep a secret?' asks Uncle Ralph.

'I want my Mammy.'

'But can you keep a secret?'

'I want to go home now.'

'This must be our special secret game. If you tell anyone I will tell your Mammy that you went in the paddling pool and something bad will happen. Now you don't want to make her cross with you do you Lorraine, so are you going to keep the secret?'

I nod my head because I don't want to upset my Mammy, not after I promised to be good.

'Do you want to be my special little girl friend?'

'I want to go home.'

'You can go home later.'

I don't like my Uncle Ralph any more; he is rude, I can see his 'thing'. Grahame's got a thing; I saw it when he was doing a wee wee. Mammy said that all boys and Mister's have things. I don't like them; I think they are horrible.

'Lie down,' says Uncle Ralph.
'I want to get dressed now.'
'Later, now lie down, that's a good girl.'

I lie down. The floor feels hard. The bare canvas is cold on my back.
'Now don't forget this is our secret.'
Water runs down Uncle Ralph's face.
I lie on the floor for a long time. My dress still lies in a crumpled heap.
I can feel something soft and warm rubbing my tummy.
I think Uncle Ralph has a cold; he is breathing funny.
.
My tummy aches. I want to go home.

I can hear someone knocking on the door.
'Uncle Ralph, it's me.'
Uncle Ralph stands up quickly, pulls up his trousers and tells me to sit up. 'Get dressed,' he says quickly.
The knocking on the door continues.
'Hurry up.'
I get dressed. My new dress is dirty and still damp and I wonder what my Mammy is going to say when she sees me.
I turn my head and can see my brother standing on the step. 'The other shop was shut,' he says.
Uncle Ralph takes the empty bottles. 'You'd better come in then,' he says crossly.

Uncle Ralph takes us to the top of our street. Grahame runs on in front.
'Don't forget about our little secret,' says Uncle Ralph, 'and you can come to the flat and see me any time you want.'

'Well you are a little muck tub,' laughs Mammy when I walk into the house, 'I can see you've had a nice time.

Chapter 4

'Mrs Tranmer your Mini has kicked the window cleaner's bucket over again.'
Diane Smith stands on our step. Diane is always telling tales.
'Did you Lorraine?' asks Mammy.
I nod my head.
'I told you last time it's naughty to kick the window cleaner's bucket over.'
'I know it is' I said.
'Well then why did you do it?'
'Because the water was really sudsy and nice.'
'Well you mustn't do it again. The window cleaner works very hard and he's a nice mister' said Mammy.
'I don't like misters any more,' I said.
Mammy sighed, 'Why on earth not?' she said.
'Cos, well I just don't.'
Mammy shakes her head and goes into the kitchen.

'I'll be a mister one day,' said Grahame.
I look up. I didn't know Grahame had been listening.
'So that means you won't like me.'
'Yes I will.'
'No you won't.'
'I will.'
'If you don't like misters then you won't like me, so why don't you like misters?'
'They make you keep secrets,' I mutter.
'Secret? Have you got a secret?'
'Yes.'
'Tell me it.'
'I can't.'
'Why?'
'Because, well because it's a secret,' I said.
'But we always tell each other all of our secrets.'
'Can't tell.'
'Why?'
'I will get into trouble.' I say, bursting into tears.
'Why, what have you done?'
I shake my head. 'Well I went into the paddling pool at the park and

Mammy said I couldn't and he said that if I tell the secret he will tell me Mammy about it and she'd be upset..'

'Who said?' asked Grahame.

'Uncle Ralph,' I stutter.

'What's the secret? It's all right, you can tell me I won't say anything about the paddling pool.'

'You promise?'

'Course I do Lorraine. I wouldn't tell on you.'

I take a deep breath. 'You remember when we went to the park with Uncle Ralph?

Well I saw Uncle Ralph's thing, he made me lay down and rubbed it on my tummy and I was bare and I felt bit a sick.'

'That's rude, you should tell Mammy,' said Grahame.

'Should I?'

'Yes, it was very rude and naughty he shouldn't have done that, anyway,' went on Grahame, 'I think Mammy already knows about the pool.'

I hear our letterbox open.

'Grahame!' shouts Colin 'Are you playing out?'.

'Coming! You must tell me Mam,' said Grahame before going out of our front door and into the street to play with his friend.

But I don't want to tell Mammy; what if something bad happens?

Chapter 5

I'm wearing my best dress again today. It is all nice and clean now. Grahame is wearing his best shirt. Mammy said we have to look our best because a mister is coming to take our photograph. I don't want to have my picture taken, I want to go out and play. Jill is also having her photograph taken and so is Colin. Jill is my best friend she lives next door to me.

Mammy sits me on the sideboard.
'Say Cheese,' says the mister.
I look down at my poorly knee where I had fallen down in the terrace.
'Smile Mini,' says Mammy, 'and sit up, come on smile, let's see your lovely white teeth.'
I look at the patterns on my best dress and remember the last time I wore it.
'Come on smile, that's a good girl, the mister wants to take your photo, and you look so pretty.'
I don't feel like smiling.
'If you give us a nice big smile I will give you one of my goodies,' says Grahame.
I make myself smile but it's not a proper smile. There is a flash of light and the picture is taken.
'Can I go out and play now?' I ask Mammy. 'I don't want to wear this dress any more, I want my blue one on.'
'I can't understand you Mini,' says Mammy, 'you used to love this dress.'
It's a very hot day. Jill is sitting on her step. She is eating a red ice lolly.
I'm very thirsty but the ice cream van has disappeared around the corner.
'Hiya Mini,' says Jill 'You coming over to play?'
I run up to Jill and sit by her side on the step. My mouth waters as I watch her licking her ice lolly.
'Jill,' I say, 'do you want to play a good game?'
'Yes,' says Jill happily.
'Well let's pretend I'm a big bad wolf and when you're not looking I gobble up your lolly.'
'Al-right,' laughs Jill.

'Well turn around then.'

Jill turns around and I take a bite of her lolly, swallow it quickly, then take a bigger bite.

Jill turns back. Her lolly has almost gone and the tiny bit that is left is melting and dripping from her fingers.

'Mammy!' shouts Jill, bursting into tears, 'that Mini has pinched my lolly.'

'You naughty girl!' shouts my Mammy who had been busy washing the windows, 'say you're sorry to Jill for being so greedy.'

I tell Jill I'm sorry but she doesn't want to play any more and just sits on her step sulking.

'You'd better go inside,' says Mammy,

I go in the house and play with my poppet doll.

'Dolls are stupid,' says Grahame.

'No they're not,' I say, pulling a cord from the doll's back, 'this one can talk.'

Grahame laughs. 'It's still stupid,'

'No it isn't.'

'Have you told me Mam the secret yet?' asks Grahame.

'No,'

'Why?'

'Because if I do Mammy will find out that I went in the mucky paddling pool and she'll be cross.'

'Mammy knows.'

'What about?'

'About you going in the pool; I told her.'

'Tell tale tit!' I shout.

'I'm not,' says Grahame, 'she asked me so I told her, anyway she didn't get mad or anything.'

'I can't tell.'

'The secret?'

'No.'

'Why? Me Mam won't chow at you.'

'I know, but something bad will happen if I tell.'

'Who told you that?'

'He did.'

'Who? Uncle Ralph?'

'Yes and I'm frightened.' I start to cry.

Grahame put his arm around me. 'There's no need to be scared,' he said. 'Don't worry, just tell your Mammy, nowt's going to happen, you'll see.'

Grahame gives me a goodie and I start to feel a bit better.

I hear the door open and Mammy walks into the room.

'Have you been crying?' she says, looking at my face.

Grahame nudges me. 'Tell her,' he whispers, 'tell her now.'

'Tell her what?' says Mammy.

'Oh, it's nothing,' I mutter.

Grahame sighs.

'Are you sure, Lorraine?' says Mammy. 'Do you want to go back out and play, it's that what's the matter?'

I nod my head.

'Well go on then, but be good,' says Mammy.

I run outside and Grahame follows me. 'You didn't tell her,' he says.

'You should tell me Mam, it's not right.'

'I want to play out,' I say.

'Will you tell her later?'

'All right.'

'Promise.'

'Yeah, I promise Grahame, I'll tell her later.'

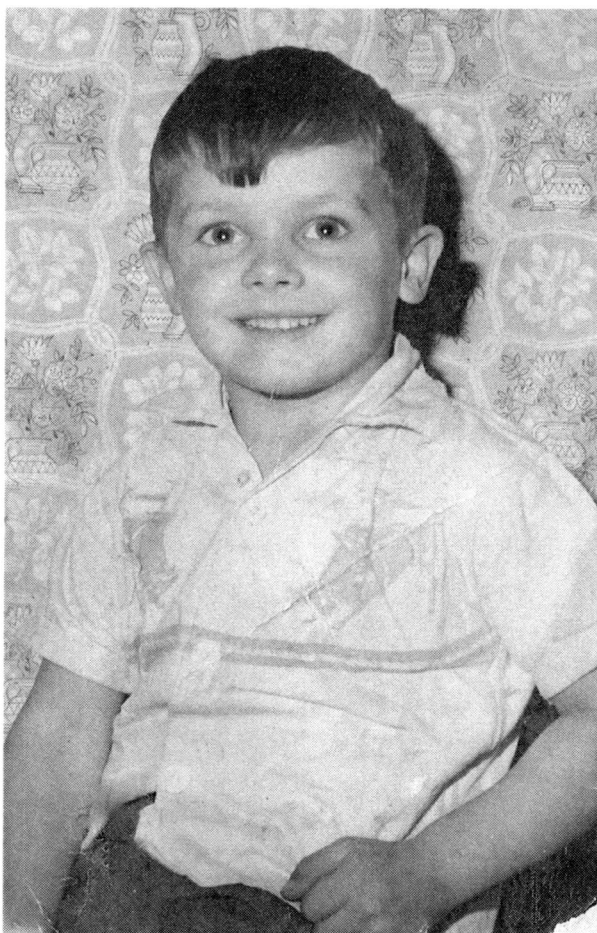

Grahame aged six

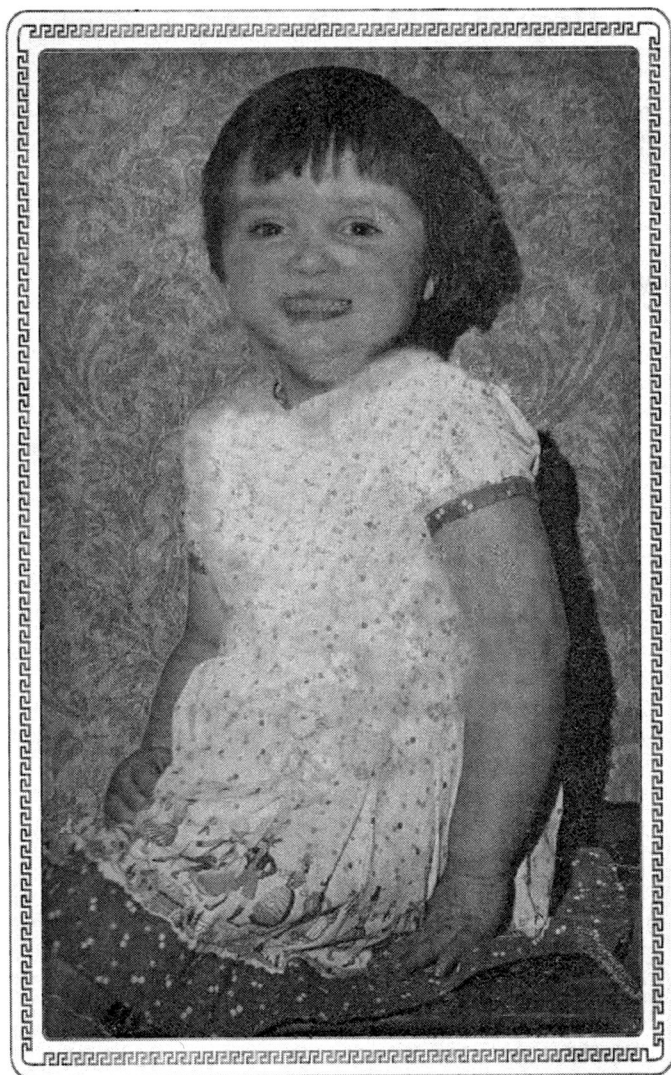

Lorraine aged five

Chapter 6

'Come on you two, up the dilly dancers,' said Mammy, 'it's time for bed.'
I pick my rag doll up which Mammy made and Grahame and I go up the stairs to our room. Mammy follows behind.

'Now do want me to sing you?' says Mammy as she tucks us up in our beds.
'Wynken Blynken and Nod,' I say as I snuggle down under the covers.
'But that's for babies,' says Grahame, 'and it's stupid.'
Ignoring Grahame Mammy begins to sing.
'Wynken Blynken and Nod one night
Sailed off in a wooden shoe
Sailed on a river of crystal light,
Into a sea of dew.'
I close my eyes while my Mammy sings.

"Where are you going and what do you wish?'
The old moon asked the three.
'We have come to fish for the herring fish
That live in this beautiful sea;
Nets of silver and gold have we!'
Said Wynken Blynken and Nod.'
Very soon I can hear Grahame snoring. Mammy carries on singing.
'All night long their nets they threw,
To the stars in their twinkling foam-
Then down from the skies came the wooden shoe
Bringing the fishermen home.
It was all so pretty a sail it seemed
As if it could not be.
And some folks thought it was a dream they'd dreamed.
Of sailing that beautiful sea.
But I shall name you the fishermen three,
Wynken Blynken and Nod.'

I sit up in bed and rub my eyes.
'Lie back down and try to sleep,' said Mammy.
'I can't.'

'Why, you like this song, come on, snuggle back down while I sing you the last bit.'

Mammy strokes my forehead and carries on singing.

'Wynken and Blynken are two little eyes,
And Nod is a little head,
And the wooden shoe that sailed the skies is a little one's trundle bed,
So close your eyes while your Mammy sings
Of wonderful sights that be
And you shall see the beautiful things,
As you rock in the misty sea,
Where the old moon rocked the fishermen three.
Wynken Blynken and Nod.

Mammy comes to the end of the song and tucks me in. 'What's the matter with you tonight? That was your favourite, you're usually fast asleep by the time I've finished it.'

'It's just that…'

'It's just what?' says Mammy, 'What's bothering you Lorraine? You haven't been yourself for a while,'

'Well it's just that I know a secret' I say. I sit up and pluck the bits of cotton from my pink eiderdown.

'What secret's that?' says Mammy.

'I don't know if I should tell you; something bad might happen.'

Mammy put her arm around me. 'You can tell me anything,' she says, 'especially something that's upsetting you. Don't worry, nothing bad will happen if you do.'

I bite hard on to my bottom lip, not knowing where to begin.

'Are you all right love?' says Mammy. 'You will feel much better when you have told me what's bothering you. Just tell me from the beginning.'

I continue pulling threads from the eiderdown. Mammy doesn't like me doing this but she doesn't say anything. 'It was when we went to park with Uncle Ralph' I say.

'Did something happen to upset you?' says Mammy.

I nod my head.

'Didn't you have a very nice time?'

'No.'

'What happened to you?'

'I slipped in the paddling pool and got all wet through. Uncle Ralph said he wouldn't tell you I went in the paddling pool because you would be very cross.'

'Is that the secret?'

'No.........When we went up some stairs to his flat and he took my clothes off I saw his thing, he told me to lay down and he rubbed it on my belly and I was a bit frightened because Grahame wasn't there. Uncle Ralph had sent him to shop with the bottles, he kept holding me real tight and I didn't like it. He said it was a secret and I was his special girl. He said that if I told anyone something horrible would happen and I was scared. He said he would tell you I went in the dirty paddling pool and and.......'   I couldn't talk any more because I started crying.

'It's all right,' says Mammy. She rocks me back and forward. 'I'm here, don't cry love, it's all right now. Maybe Uncle Ralph's trousers had fallen down by accident and his thing came out. Don't worry love, no one's going to hurt you.'

'Aren't you cross with me Mammy?' I say in between sobs.

'No love, I'm not cross with you,' says Mammy,

'But I went in the paddling pool,' I mutter.

'It doesn't matter about that,' she says as she lays me down and tucks me in again. 'I'll sit by your side until you fall sleep,' she says softly, 'don't worry, I won't let anyone hurt you ever again.'

I close my eyes feeling much better.

After that we never saw Uncle Ralph again.

Chapter 7

'Pay attention Lorraine! You're not listening to the story, in fact I
don't think you have listened to any of it, have you?'
I look away from the window. Miss Barret was right; I hadn't.

I'm so happy because after school we're going to light the big fire
and set off our fireworks. Mammy said that this year I can hold the
sparklers all by myself.
Everyone down our street has been helping to build the bonfire
which is on bombed out buildings. My Dad said that bombed
buildings are where the houses were bombed a long time ago when
there was a war. I'm not allowed to play there but the bigger kids
do. Sometimes the Seaton Street gang steal wood from our fire and
put it on to theirs. But the Symons Street gang take it back. The
gangs run through the passages which cut through the streets.

The long school day comes to an end everyone is chattering
excitedly.

Grahame has made a Mr Guy Fawkes. He has a very ugly face
with a horrible snarling mouth. He's sitting at the bottom of our
stairs dressed in a pair of my Dad's old trousers and shirt.

'Penny for the guy, penny for the guy.'
'He's a nice guy, did you make him yourself?'
'Yes Mrs, I did,' says Grahame proudly.
The grey haired woman stands on her doorstep rummaging in her
purse. 'Now let me see, what I can let you have?' she says. Smiling,
she gives Grahame a threepenny bit.
'Now off you go,' she says, 'and enjoy the bonfire.'
'Thank-you,' said Grahame, 'we will.'
We push the old pram with the guy sitting proudly in it on to the
next house.
'Penny for the guy, penny for the guy,' says Grahame the moment
the door is opened.
Without saying a word the man delves deep into his pocket and
gives Grahame a shiny brown penny.
'Thanks Mister,' says Grahame.

The bonfire is lovely. It's the biggest one I have ever seen. We watch the fireworks and then later on we sit around the fire singing.
'Bonfire night, bonfire night, all is bright, two little angels covered in shite' sing the big kids. We all laugh and join in with the singing. All too soon the night has come to an end and it's time to go home to bed.
'That was the biggest bonfire I've ever seen.' I say as I keep in step with Grahame.
'Yeah it was Mini,' says Grahame proudly, 'it was much bigger then Seaton Street's fire.'

After having a wash and putting on my nightie I lay back on the couch and close my eyes, trying to picture the lovely fire works and bonfire.
'Oh look, she's fallen asleep,' I hear Mammy say.
'She's enjoyed herself; she never stopped smiling all night' says my Dad.
'Do you think she's forgotten about that Ralph?'
'I hope so,' says my Dad.
I feel my Mammy lift me up. I keep my eyes closed and pretend to be asleep while she carries me up to bed.

That night I had my first bad dream.

Chapter 8

I'm lying on the couch. My head feels hot and my chest hurts. Mammy said I can stay off school and she has bought me a bottle of lucozade. It's all bubbly and fizzy and makes my nose tickle when I drink it. Mrs next door sat with me while Mammy went to the telephone box at the top of our street to ring the doctor. When she comes back she makes a cup of tea and her and Mrs next door sit looking at me and talking.
'She does look poorly,' says Mrs next door.
Mammy sighs loudly. 'I've been up all night with her,' she says
'You say she had a nightmare too.'

'Yes, she was screaming her little head off,' says Mammy.

'That'll be her temperature,' says Mrs next door.

Mrs next door's voice fades in the distance.

'Wake up love, the doctor's here,' I hear Mammy say.

I struggle to sit up. The doctor takes something out of his black bag.

'He's just going to listen to your chest with his stethoscope.'

Mammy tries to lift up my vest. I lie back down and put the cover over my head.
'Come on love,' says Mammy as she gently removes the cover. 'It won't hurt you.'
I lie on the couch with my eyes closed tightly. The stethoscope feels cold on my skin.
I want to cry. I don't like the doctor and I don't like being poorly.
I keep my eyes closed until I hear the doctor leave the house.
'You were a silly girl,' says my Mam. 'The doctor wasn't going to hurt you.'
'I didn't like him,' I mumble.
'Why ever not?'
'Dunno, I just didn't.'

Later on I hear my Mam tell my Dad that I have a bad chest.

My Mammy tucks me in to bed. She's just given me some yellow medicine. It tastes nice, a bit like bananas. She said it will make me feel better.

I lie in my bed counting to myself, trying hard to stay awake, afraid that the bad dream I had last night will come back. But my eyes feel hot and prickly and I don't remember reaching thirty before my eyes close.

I'm running, running faster and faster. I know he is behind me, he will catch me soon, I can hear him breathing. My tummy aches and my legs feel all wobbly like jelly and I know I can't run any more.
I fall to the ground. I open my mouth to scream, no noise comes out but I can hear my heart beating louder and louder. His hot breath is on my face. I bite my bottom lip until I can taste blood.
I hear my Mammy calling my name. She sounds like she is coming from a long, long way away.
'Lorraine, Lorraine are you all right? You have fallen out of bed.'
I open my eyes. My Mammy holds me in her arms and the bad man has gone.

I look around my bedroom; everything is the same.
'It was just a nasty dream,' says Mammy. 'It's all right, nothing's going to hurt you, I'm here now.'

I sit by the side of my bed and watch as Mammy puts on the clean dry sheets.
'Don't get upset, it was only a little accident,' she says.

'Can I sleep in your bed? I feel poorly.'
Mammy smiles as she feels my forehead. 'Just for tonight then,' she says.
My Dad goes down the stairs to sleep on the settee and I snuggle in beside my Mammy.
Very soon it is morning. I can hear Mammy getting Grahame up for school. The rain pelts down on the window. I pull the blankets right up to my neck. It's nice and warm in Mammy's bed and I'm glad that I don't have to go to school in the rain.

Mammy gives me my medicine and lays me on the settee. I've just had a chucky egg for my breakfast. It was nice and runny. It feels nice when there's just me and Mammy, and I hope I don't have to go back to school for a long, long time.

I smile and watch from my place on the settee while Mammy does the ironing. She's getting very fat and holds her tummy all the time. Perhaps, I tell myself, perhaps she has had too many sweets off Mrs Bailoid's penny tray.

I stayed off school for a full week and a half before the doctor said that I was a lot better and could go back. I didn't want to go back to school, I wanted to stay at home with Mammy, but Grahame said that if I didn't a kid catcher would come and get me. I didn't want the kid catcher to catch me so I told Mammy I wanted to return to school the very next day.

Chapter 9

Our cat has had kittens, six little black and white ones.
'Don't pick them up Mini, because if you do Tiddles will get upset and she might eat them' says Janet, a girl who lives at top of our street.

'It's true,' said Mammy, peering down into the box of kittens. 'Cats, well, they sometimes get jealous you see.'

'We can hold them when their eyes are open,' said Grahame wisely. 'It should be all right then.'

'You ought to have drowned them,' said Mrs next door who had popped in for a cup of tea.   'Old Mrs Watson will do it for you. It'll only cost you few coppers, she's all right she is, she must have drowned hundreds of litters in her time.'

I look up horrified.

'That's bloody cruel!' shouts Grahame.
'Don't swear Grahame,' says my Mammy, giving Mrs next door a dirty look at the same time.

'Why the streets are full of stinking stray cats,' says Mrs next door. 'Best thing to do if you ask me owt.'

'Nobody's asking you,' says Janet, 'so stop upsetting the bairns.'

'No need to be so cheeky,' says Mrs next door, 'I don't know who you think you are talking to me like that; you're only a snotty nosed kid yourself.'

'I'm fourteen,' says Janet, 'old enough to see that the bairns are getting upset so you want to shut your m...'

Mammy held her hands up. 'That's enough!' she shouts. 'I'm not having you arguing in my house, so we'll have no more of it.'

'Well, I'll have to be off now anyway,' says Mrs next door, standing up to leave. 'Bye Jean.' As Mrs next door turns her back Janet puts out her tongue.

I giggle. I like Janet, she's funny.
'The wicked old bugger,' says Janet as the front door closes.

The kittens grow bigger every day and so does my Mammy's tummy. She's got that fat she can hardly bend over.

*****

'Get up,' says my dad, 'you're going out with Yasmin and Annette.'
Yasmin and Annette were two big girls who lived down our terrace.
We often go swimming with them.

'Where are we going Dad?' asks Grahame.

'To the pictures,' said my dad. 'You can go to the ABC and watch the cartoons. Now come on, let's have you both dressed.'

I was so excited. 'The cartoons!' I say, jumping up and down.

'Shush,' says my daddy. 'Don't wake your Mammy up. She isn't very well, she's sleeping in the front room.'

Mammy had been sleeping in the front room for a couple of weeks now. My dad had put her a bed up in there, 'you will be warmer down here love,' he had said. 'It will be better for you when the time comes.'

'What time Dad?' I ask.

'Never you mind,' my Dad had said. 'I was talking to your mother.'

About ten minuets later we set off for the pictures.
Yasmin holds my hand tightly all the way. She isn't her usual chatty self and keeps reminding me that I must be a good girl for my Mammy.
'Is Mammy poorly?' I ask, thinking about the bed downstairs and having   to   keep   warm.'
'No, not really,' said Yasmin, 'you just have to be a good girl, that's

all.'

We sit in the front row. Grahame's laughing at Tom and Jerry but all I can think about is my Mammy, my Dad's worried face and that bed downstairs in the front room.

After what seems like ages the cartoons come to an end. 'Thank god for that,' I mutter to myself. 'Now I can go home back to Mammy.'

I stand up to leave. 'Sit back down Mini,' says Yasmin with a big smile on her face. 'We're going to watch it again.'

'Oh great!' shouts Grahame as he settles back in his seat.

The cartoons seem to go on for ever. My ice lolly melts in my hand and my tummy aches. The kids sitting in the front row are laughing loudly but I'm not taking much notice of anything. I just want to go home.

Finally the cartoons come to an end once again. We leave the cinema and make our way to the bus stop.

'That was great,' says Grahame.

Yasmin looks down at me. 'Did you enjoy the cartoons Mini?' she asks.

I shrug my shoulders.

'She's stupid,' says Grahame, 'all girls are stupid.'

'No they are not,' says Yasmin, 'Mini's just tired, that's all.'

Annete put out her hand and the bus comes to a standstill at the bus stop.

We sit at the back.

As we walk down our terrace I can see Mrs Carte and Mrs next door stood on their doorsteps.

'Hiya me little cockbod,' said Mrs Lyle Carter as I pass her. Mrs Carter calls all the kids 'cockbod'.

Mrs next door looks across at me. She's smiling and nodding her head.

The first thing I see when I enter our house are doctors' bags lining the narrow hallway.

My dad peeps his head around the door.

'Where's my Mam?' shouts Grahame.

My dad puts his finger to his lips. 'Hush,' he says, 'your Mam's gone shopping down Charles Street.' His face then breaks out into a huge grin. 'Go in the front room,' he says, 'but be quiet.'

My Mammy is sitting propped up by the pillows. She looks happy but sort of tired.

'Come and give me cuddle,' she says.

I give Mammy a big hug and a kiss. Mammy then points to the other side of the bed. Perched on top of a small chest of drawers I notice a blue baby carry cot.

'Go and meet your new baby brother,' she says.

I peer inside the carry cot. A tiny baby with his eyes wide open is lying there.

'His name's Michael and he's only one hour old' says Mammy.

'Oh Mammy he's lovely, are we going to keep him?'

'Yes,' says Mammy, 'he's ours.'

'Where did he come from?'

'The nurse brought him for us this morning,' said my dad who had come into the room and was standing by the door.

'Did she fetch him in one of those black bags that's in the passage?'

'Aye,' says my dad smiling and nodding his head, 'she did.'

I gaze back into the carry cot and look at my little brother's tiny hands. He isn't much bigger than my baby doll. Grahame stands by my side. 'I would rather have had a rabbit,' he says, wiping his runny nose on the sleeve of his jumper.

'Oh Mammy, Mam, can I hold him?' I ask.

'Not just now love, but you can later' she says.

'Let your Mammy have a little rest now Mini,' says my dad.

Slowly I leave the bedroom.

'Is me Mam all right?' asks Grahame.

'She's fine,' says my dad, 'just a bit tired.'

'Why is she tired?' I ask. 'Is she poorly?'

My Dad shook his head. 'No, she's not ill.'

'Then why is she tired?'

'W...l...l,' stammers my dad, 'it's just that babies, well they make you tired sometimes. And your Mammy needs her rest so that she can look after it.'

'Can I go out and play then?' I ask.

'If you promise to stay in the terrace,' says my dad.

'Oh but Dad, I want to go and see my Aunty Maud.'

'No, stay in terrace,' says my dad.

'All right then Dad,' I say as I close the door behind me.

Jill is sitting on the fence.

'Jill, Jill! I shout running up to her. 'We've got a new baby. The nurse brought him in her black bag this morning and....a n d his name is Michael.'

'I know,' said Jill, 'our Mam told me ages ago.'

'Oh,' I say quietly.

'Do you wanna go and play on bomb buildings?' asks Jill.

'No, I'm not allowed. I gotta stay in the terrace.'

'Well, I'm allowed, so there,' says Jill, sticking out her tongue .

'Shall we play at hopscotch then?'

'No,' says Jill, 'I'm going to play on bomb buildings.'

'It's not fair' I mutter as I hop onto the numbered squares.

I notice my grandad as he shuffles up our terrace. He is a very, very old man and has a crooked back and a bad cough. He is always holding his tummy and saying his 'bowels are bad.' He lives at the top of our terrace. His house is very dark and smoky. He sits in the back room most of the day spitting into the fire. My Mam says he also has a bad chest. I run up to him. 'Grandad, I've got a little brother,' I say.

'How's our Jean?' says my Grandad without looking up.

'Oh, me Mam's fine, she's just having a little rest.'

My Grandad nods his head and goes on his way, shuffling up our terrace.

He's strange is my Grandad, and I don't think he ever has a bath because he keeps his coal in his tin bath in the front room. Maybe that's why he smells a bit.

I don't remember my Grandma. My Mam told me she died when I was just a tiny baby.

I have another Grandma though, that's my dad's Mam. She lives in Hedon and sometimes we go and see her on a Saturday. She lives at the bottom of a lane in a little wooden house that has roses growing around her door. I love going to see my Grandma. Her garden is very big and she has lots of apple trees and a pear tree. The only thing I don't like about my Grandma's is her toilet. It isn't a proper toilet with a chain. It is just a big drum inside a box with a seat on it . My Mam says it's called an earth toilet.

Our terrace is empty now. All the kids are playing in the street.

Feeling lonely and bored I go back into our house.
My dad and our Grahame are sat watching the Olympic games on
the television.

'I'm hungry Dad, what's for dinner?' I ask.
'Hush!' says my Dad, his eyes not leaving the television.
'Grahame's going to the fish shop soon so go back out and play.'
'Can I go back in the front room to see me Mam?'
'No, your Mam is asleep.'
'Can I play in the street with the other kids?'
'No, I've told you to stay in the terrace.'
'But why can't I play…'
'Just do as your told Mini, that's a good lass.'

I walk by the front room and quietly open the door. My Mam is
sitting up in bed with the new baby in her arms. She smiles at me
and I sit on the side of the bed.
'Would you like to hold your little brother?' she asks.
'Oh yes Mammy.'
'Sit back then,' says Mammy.
I rest my back on the bed head and my Mam puts little Michael on
my knees.
I look into his little round face and rock him gently back and forth.
A warm feeling washes over me and I want to cry. My little brother
looks up at me as if to say, 'well I'm here now, whether you like it
or not.'

Chapter 10

'Come on Lorraine, get your hat and coat on,' says Mammy.
'Are we going shopping?'
'We're going to for a walk and popping into the baby shop to get your little brother a new helmet.'
'Can I choose it Mammy?
'Yes, now get your coat on, it's a bit chilly.'
'That's not fair,' said Grahame, 'I want to pick it, she'll pick something sissy.'
'You can both choose it, now hurry up,' says my Mam.

'Can I push the pram Mammy?' I ask as we make our way down our street.
'All right,' says my Mam, 'but only until we get to the road.'
I can hardly see over the pram hood but I feel sort of all grown up as I walk along.
Jill has got her doll's pram out. I just smile at her and nod my head as I proudly walk by her pushing my little brother in his pram.
We reach the road and my Mam takes the handlebars and I hold on at the side of the pram as we make our way down Charles Street. Grahame runs on in front.
The baby shop is about halfway down.   My Mam parks the pram near the window and lifts little Michael up. The bell rings as we enter the shop and a lady sitting behind the counter amidst countless balls of wool and baby clothes smiles at us.
'Good morning, can I help you?' she says as she admires my baby brother.
I clear my throat.   'Yes,' I say, feeling very important, 'we would like a helmet for my little brother.'
'I see,' says the lady. 'Now we have some very nice ones here.'
The lady puts a box on the counter containing tiny knitted helmets.
'This one's a nice one,' she says picking up a cream lace one.
'No, that's too sissy,' says Grahame.
'Well how about this one then?' says the lady.
Me Mam puts the white helmet near Michael's face but it looks a bit too big.
'No, that doesn't look right,' I say.
After looking through the rest of the helmets in the box Grahame and I decide that none of them are really suitable for *our* little

brother. They're either too big for him, or the colour isn't right, they are too sissy or they just don't suit him. Sighing, the lady puts the box back under the counter and we leave the shop. We walk the full length of Charles Street and enter another shop. We don't like the helmets in there either, so my Mam says we can go and have a look at the shops down Beverley Road.

After walking down Beverley Road for some time we find a shop which sells baby clothes. The first three helmets we see aren't what we want, then the lady shows us a little turquoise one. We try it on our little Michael. He looks really bonny in it, the colour seems to match his eyes.

"Is that one good enough for him?' says my Mam.

Grahame and I nod our heads.

'Well thank God for that,' says my Mam.

The lady wraps the new helmet up in tissue paper and we proudly leave the shop.

One year later

Chapter 11

It's nearly the end of the long school holiday. I won't be in the Infant school when we go back, I will be a Junior.

Because of my bad chest my Mam and Dad have decided that I must go to a different school, so I will no longer be going to the little school at the top of our street I will be getting the bus and going all the way to Fifth Avenue school which is in North Hull. North Hull is far way from the factories which belch out all the filth and smog out for people to breathe in.

I'm looking forward to going to the new school because it has a field to play games in and not just a small concrete playground. I can't help feeling sad though because I know I will miss my friends.

The new school day finally arrives. My Mam walks with me to the bus stop at the top of Beverly Road. Denise is also going to Fifth Avenue school. Together we get on the bus. My Mam waves to me but I pretend I haven't seen her as I sit down and pay the conductor my fare. As the bus speeds up the road all sorts of thoughts run round in my head. 'What if I don't like it? The work may be too hard, the other kids might hate me, what if the teachers are horrible?'

After some time the bus stops outside the school. I stand up. My stomach aches and my legs have gone all wobbly. My mouth is dry and I want to be sick and I wish with all my heart that I was still in the infant school down Fountain Road.

'Good morning girls,' said Mrs Grace, my teacher. 'We have a new girl and her name is Lorraine and I want all of you to make her welcome to our school.'

I stand at the front of the class feeling sick and wanting the ground to open up and swallow me. Mrs Grace smiles at me then points to an empty desk at the front of the class and tells me to sit down. I can feel the eyes of the other girls watching me curiously as I sit on the edge of the chair. Mrs Grace hands out some new exercise books and gives me a separate piece of paper with sums written on them which she asks me to do. I pick up my pencil and begin to do them. The sums are very easy and I soon have them finished.

'That's just a test,' says a girl behind me, 'the work gets much harder then that.'

'Be quite child!' barks Mrs Grace, 'I'll have no talking in the class.'
The morning soon passes and the big bell goes to signal it's time for
playtime, or break as it is called in this school.
'You may leave your desks but no running,' says Mrs Grace.
I stand up slowly and follow the gang of girls outside to the
playground. The field is only used for P.E. and games, and I feel
very disappointed about this as I had looked forward to playing in it
and feeling the soft grass beneath my feet.

I stand alone in the corner of the playground hoping that soon the
whistle will be blown and I can go back inside.
Four girls walk up to me.
'Hey new girl!' one of them shouts. 'Are you old enough to be in our
school?'
I nod my head.
'How old are you?' asks another girl.
'I'm seven and a bit,' I mutter.
'Well you're tiny for your age,' says the girl 'you look like you
belong in the infants' school.'
'Do you wanna play with us?'
'Yes,' I reply.
'Well come and turn the skipping rope with Julie while we skip.'
Smiling, I follow the girls to the middle of the playground.

'One two three,
Me Mother caught a flea.
She put it in the teapot,
To make a cup of tea.
The flea jumped out,
Me Mother gave a shout,
And down came me Dad,,
With his shirt hanging out.'
Sang the girls while Julie and me turned the skipping rope. The line
of girls took their turns to jump in and out of it.
When all the girls had had their turn a fat fair haired girl looks at
me. 'It's your turn,' she says.
I hand the rope to anther girl who then begins to turn it.
I stand by the side of the rope.
'Come on then, jump!' shouts Julie.
I tried with all my might but I couldn't for the life off me jump over
the twisting twirling rope.

'She can't even skip' says a girl.
'She's useless,' mutters another.
At that moment and to my relief the whistle is blown.
'Will you all quietly form your lines and make your way back to
your classrooms?' says the teacher.   As   I walk back into the
classroom I can hear Julie and her friend sniggering behind me.
'That new girl's stupid, she can't even skip' I hear Julie mutter.
Feeling sad and ashamed I sit down at my desk.

The rest of the day slowly passes. I don't like this new school very
much with the strange giggling girls.   I miss Fountain Road school,
my friends, and even some of the boys.
At last it's time to go home.

The bus is taking forever to arrive and the rain falls down and seeps
into my coat.   There is no shelter at the bus stop so I stand there
praying for the bus to hurry up.
The bus finely arrives. I sit near the window soaking wet with my
teeth chattering.

****

'What's your new school like?' asks my Mam.
'It's great Mam,' I lie.
'Did you make any new friends?'
'Yeah, lots,' I say, trying to smile.
Michael is sitting in his high chair. I walk up to him and ruffle his
white hair.
'Can I go out and play?'
'Yes, but get changed out of your school clothes.'
Sighing, I change into my playing out clothes.

Jill is sitting on her step.
'What's Fifth Ave' school like then?' she says.
'It's horrible,' I mutter.
'I think you're lucky going to a school with no daft boys in it and a
playing field.'
'Well, I don't like it and I wish I was back at Fountain Road school.'
'Do you wanna play at houses?' says Jill, holding her doll.
'Yeah, but I wanna be the Mam' I say.
'You can't be the Mam, it's my doll, anyway I'm bigger than you.'

I don't want to play with you then!' I cry.

I slam back into my house wishing I wasn't small for my age, and most of all wishing I didn't have to go back to that horrible school in the morning.

Chapter 12

'Lorraine, I've got something to tell you,' said my Mam, looking very happy and pleased with herself.

I shift from foot to foot. 'What is it? Tell me Mam, oh please tell me.'

'I already know,' smiles Grahame.

'Well,' says my Mam, 'in seven days' time we are going to move to a new house.'

'A new house?'

'Yes, well, it's not really a house, it's a little bungalow,' smiles my Mam. 'It's near your Gran's.'

'It's down the lane,' says Grahame jumping up and down, 'in Hedon.'

'The lane!'

'Yeah, and we'll have a big garden. Oh, it's going to be great,' says Grahame.

'Will I be going to a different school?'

'Yeah of course you will, stupid.'

'Don't call her stupid,' says my Mam. 'You will be going to the same school your dad went to when he was young. 'It's a lovely little school and you'll make some new friends.'

Excitement bubbles up inside me. I can hardly believe it's true. I love it down the lane where there are no factories and the air smells fresh and clean.

'Well what do you think?' My Mam takes one look at my face and knows then that I feel as happy as she is.

My Mam sits back in her chair, contented. 'The spring's a lovely time to move house,' she sighs. 'A perfect time for new beginnings.'

Chapter 13

'Do you want to go to see your Gran while I do some work on the new house?' asks my dad.
I nod my head excitedly and my dad picks me up and sits me in the middle of the handcart. I giggle as my dad pulls the handcart with ease down the street. A group of kids wave and smile as we go by. I smile back proudly. He's very strong, is my dad.
Very soon we leave the streets behind.
I giggle to myself, unable to contain my excitement.
My dad turns around. He is smiling all over his face. 'Are you enjoying the ride me little lass?' he says.
'Yeah, it's great.'
I sit in the middle of the handcart feeling like the Queen of Sheba.

After some time the factories are replaced with green fields. I can see baby lambs and cows. It's so different to looking from a bus window. Hugging myself I take in the fresh air. My dad turns around to face me. 'We're nearly there,' he says.
He then points to a sign at the side of the road. 'That says Hedon,' he says proudly.
'Are we really here Dad,' I say, hardly daring to believe it, for I must have been sitting on that handcart for hours and my backside has gone all numb.
'Aye,' says my dad, 'we're here.'
We pass a shop and a row of houses with gardens at the front.
Very soon we come to the lane.
When we reach the top of the lane my dad lifts me from the handcart. 'You can walk from here,' he says.
'Hiya Doug,' says a woman walking by, 'this your young 'un then.'
'Aye, she is an all, Mrs Dovey,' says my dad.
The old lady looks me up and down. 'Well there's no need to tell me that Doug, she's the image of you when you was a bairn.' Mrs Dovey smiles at me then turns to my dad. ' Your Mam tells me you're moving back down the lane.' she says.
'Aye we are,' says my dad, 'in a couple of days.'
'I'm pleased for you lad.' Old Mrs Dovey walks on, smiling to herself.
I try my hardest not to laugh. It seems funny hearing someone call

my dad 'lad'.

I skip along looking at the funny little wooden houses with the big gardens. We turn a corner near a field.
'That's Doby's field,' says my dad 'and you see that big tree there,' he says, pointing to the biggest tree I had ever seen.
'Yes Dad.'
'Well I use to climb that when I was a lad.'
'Right to the very top!'
'Yes,' says my dad, 'I did.'
I look up to the big tree and the branches seem to touch the sky.
'There're loads and loads of trees and fields here,' says my dad.
'Plenty of places for you to play. It will be different to being down that street you know.' My dad smiles to himself. 'You can walk for miles and not see a soul; it's great.'
'But what about the cows, Dad?'
'Oh cows won't hurt you; they're gentle animals.' My dad laughs and we go on our way.

'What is the number of our new house Dad?' I ask.
'The houses have names instead of numbers,' says my dad.
'What's the name of our new house then Dad?'
'It's called Mayfield Villas and it's a lovely little place.'
'I can't wait to see it,' I say, hugging myself.
'You're not seeing it today Lorraine, it will spoil the surprise on moving day, because,' went on my dad, 'moving days are special days. So you're going to stay with your Gran today while I get it ready for us all.'
'Dad?'
'Yes Love.'
'What do they call me Gran's house?'
'Well your Grandma's house is called Nevilda but they're not houses, they're called bungalows because they don't have any stairs.'
'N e v i l d a,' I say. 'That's a funny name for a house, I mean a bungalow,'
'It's called Nevilda,' says my dad, 'because it once belonged to a couple called Nevil and Hilda.'
'Oh, I see.'
'And your Great Aunt, well she lives in a bungalow called Glandown.'
My dad then points to bungalows as we walk along. 'That one's

called Rosedene,' he says, pointing to a small green bungalow. He
then points to the other side of the road, 'and that one there's called
Dunroamin.'
He points to many others as we walk along, telling me their names.
I look at the small bungalows. Most of them are made of wood.
They look so different from the back to back houses down the street.

As we walk further down the lane I can see my Gran waiting for us
near her garden. She is smiling and waving.
My Gran's house smells of apples and flowers. She is always baking
and has a big oven near her fire. It has little doors in it which she
polishes every day.
I love going down the lane to see my Gran, and although I know I
will miss all my cousins and friends down the street, I am still very
happy to be going to live down the lane and starting a new school.

Chapter 14

I open my eyes as the spring sunshine filters through the window. I know that there is something different about today. But it doesn't come to me straight away what it is.

I can hear my Mam and Dad talking in their bedroom.

'What time did you say the van will be here Jean?' I hear my dad say.

'Just after dinner,' says my Mam with an edge of excitement in her voice.

'Van, what van,' I muse sleepily.

Suddenly I realise what they are talking about and what's so special about today. I sit bolt upright in my bed, smiling to myself, for today's the day I have been waiting for, today is moving day.

I glance across at Grahame's bed. He is still sleeping with his mouth wide open, catching flies. I look around our bedroom as though for the first time and find it hard to take in that tomorrow morning I will be waking up somewhere else.

I look up, noticing the pink and blue blobs of cotton stuck to the ceiling, and I smile sadly to myself as I remember me and my brother's game of pulling threads with our mouths from our pink and blue candlewick bedspreads and spitting them up to the ceiling.

I hear the stairs creaking as my Mam and Dad go down them and I think how odd it will seem living in a house that has no stairs.

Quickly I get out of bed dress and go down the stairs.

I don't eat much breakfast.

'Now you can have a little wash and go to Bailods for some goodies' says my Mam, filling up the kettle. We wait for it to boil, then my Mam fills the blue plastic bowl with water. I watch as the steam rises up to the ceiling. My Mam adds the cold water and then gives me the soap and flannel to wash my hands and face.

'Now I want you to be a real good lass today,' she says, 'because we are going to be very busy.'

'Mam, Mam,' says Grahame who has just come down the stairs, 'can I go to the new house in the removal van?'

'No,' says my Mam, 'you will be better going on the bus with our Lorraine and little Michael.'

'All right,' sighs Grahame, a bit disappointed.

After my rather hasty wash my Mam gives me a threepenny bit.
'Now off you go to Bailods and get yourself some sweets' she says.
'And try to keep out of the way a bit.'
I give my Mam a kiss and go out of the front door and into the
terrace.

Clutching my threepenny bit I enter Bailods shop.
'Hiya lovie,' says Mrs Bailod, 'I suppose you'll be wanting
something off the penny tray.
'Yes please Mrs Bailod.'
I stand and watch as Mrs Bailod takes out the large silver tray from
beneath the counter.
'It's moving day today,' I say as I look at the goodies on the tray.
'I know,' says Mrs Bailod. 'You're moving to Hedon, aren't you?'
I nod my head happily.
'You're a lucky lass,' clucks Mrs Bailod.
'Me Mam says they're all posh in Hedon,' says Dianne Porter who
had just come in the shop, 'and that you won't like it very much.'
'Off course she's going to like it,' says Mrs Bailod, giving Dianne a
long look.
'But they're all real posh and talk all la de da like,' says Dianne.
'Well I'm sure Mini can be posh if she wants to,' says Mrs Bailod.
I choose a packet of refreshers, and two bars of toffee from the
tray.
I give Mrs Bailod my threepenny bit and walk towards the door.
'Tara Mini,' says Mrs Bailoid 'and don't worry, it's lovely in Hedon.'
'Bye Mrs Bailoid,' I say quietly, no longer quite so excited.
I walk towards our terrace and I can see the big removal van parked
outside.
I stand and watch as two men load furniture into the van.
Some of our neighbours are standing on their steps. I can hear
snatches of their conversation as I walk by.
'Going to live in Hedon.'
'Must have come into money.'

'Maybe had a win at bingo.'
On seeing me pass the neighbours quickly change the subject.
'I've got me name at the corporation, I think we'll be off to either
Greafield or Longhill when they pull these houses down.'
'They should have been pulled ages ago' says a grey haired woman.
'The demolition order was years ago.'

A gang of kids stand round the removal van. I wander up to them.
'Is it you that's flitting today?' asks Colin, a boy who lives down our
terrace.
'Yes,' I say, 'but I will see you all again because I will still be
coming down the street to see me Grandad and me Auntie Maud and
Uncle Bill' I say.
'Yeah, but you wont be in our gang any more,' says Colin.
'Why not?'
'Because you won't be one of us any more,' says Colin.
Feeling a bit sad, I walk away.

Our house looks funny with no furniture. The front room seems so
big.
I go up the stairs.
'Come on Lorraine!' shouts my Mam, 'We're going to catch the
twenty to seventy nine bus to Hedon.'
I take one last look at our bedroom and slowly walk towards the
door.

'Just think,' smiles Grahame as we climb on to the bus, 'it won't be
long and we'll be seeing our new house for the first time.'
'I'll miss me friend's though,' I say, still feeling a little sad.
'But you'll make new friends,' says Grahame 'and just think, we
will be living down the lane for ever and ever. It will be great.'
The street seems a long way away now and I sit back in my seat, my
excitement returning.

The bus stops outside Johnson's garage which is at top of the lane.
'We're here!' shouts Grahame.
We all get off the bus and we make our way down the lane.
'What's our new house like Mam?' says Grahame
'You'll see soon,' says my Mam.
We pass Dobey's field and I show Grahame the big tree my dad
used to climb when he was young.
'I'm going to climb that tree,' he says. 'I'm going to climb lots and
lots of trees. And I'm gonna collect birds eggs and make dens, go
fishing in drains, and, and I'm gonna explore, and I'm gonna...'
'All right, steady on,' says my Mam, smiling.
'Well, it's great down here,' sighs Grahame.
'Yeah, it is it's lovely,' I say as I breathe in the fresh air and listen to
the birds singing.

A big white horse is tethered on some overgrown land.
'Oh look Mam,' I say, 'isn't he lovely?'
My Mam doesn't say anything but she just pushes Michael faster in his tansad until she has gone by the horse.
I think my Mam's afraid of horses.
Michael is laughing as my Mam bumps his tansad over the bumpy lane.
We are about half way to the bottom of the lane when my Mam stops.
'We're here,' she says, pointing to a small gate. The gate has a piece of wood nailed to it with the name 'Mayfield Villas' written on it in faded fancy joined up writing.
Grahame opens the gate and we go down a long path which has a hedge on both sides.
At the end of the path stands our new home.
'There it is, look,' says my Mam, 'isn't it bonny?'
'Oh great, we're on the drain bank!' shouts Grahame jumping up and down.
I look at our new home for the first time, and it is so bonny. It is made of wood and painted a nice green colour. And the garden, well, I can't believe my eyes because the garden seems enormous and overgrown. At the side of the garden stands a tree.
'Your dad will put a swing up on that tree for you' says my Mam.
'I'm going to build a tree house,' smiles Grahame, looking up into the branches.
Inside the bungalow smells a little bit musty, and cobwebs have gathered in the corner of the room. The removal men had already got there, there are boxes all over the floor.
'It needs a bit of a spring clean,' laughs my Mam.
'But not to worry, I'll soon have it as bright as a new pin.'
The bungalow has a kitchen, a living room and two bedrooms.
'That's your bedroom,' says my Mam, pointing to a door at the side of the room.
My Mam follows me and Grahame into the room.
'It will look nice when we have decorated it,' she says.
I look around the room.
'That's your bed,' says my Mam, pointing to a small bed beneath the window.
'And soon your dad's going to put a partition up.'
'Oh great,' says Grahame, 'it'll be like having my own room.'
My Mam turns to Grahame. ' Yes, but soon you will have to share

with little Michael' she says.

'That will be fun,' says Grahame as he leaves the room.

I walk over to my little bed and look out of the window. I can see cows grazing in the meadow across the drain. For someone used to looking out at a small square back yard and back to back houses it really is a pretty sight.

Chapter 15

Our new home cost three hundred and fifty pounds. As it was such a lot of money Mrs Louise, the lady my dad bought it from, had agreed to let him pay for it in weekly payments.
Mrs Louise lives down the lane in a bungalow called THE BAYS. I think Mayfield Villas used to be her sister's bungalow.
On our way to our new school we call in on Mrs Louise's to make the first payment.
We knock on her door and Mrs Louise smiles and lets us in.
She gives Grahame, Michael and me a biscuit. 'Do you want a cup of tea Jean?' she says.
'Well I'm just taking Grahame and Lorraine to school,' says my Mam. 'It's their first day today.'
'Come back later then.' Mrs Louise takes a tin from a small cupboard. She opens it and as my Mam passes her the money she writes something down in a black book.

My new school is a lot smaller than my last one. My Mam drops us off at the gate as she had put our name down the previous day.
'Now mind your manners,' she said before she left.
The teacher rings the school bell and the kids all stop still in their tracks.
'Are you the new children?' asks the teacher with the bell.
Grahame nods his head. I try to hold his hand but he won't let me.
'My name is Mrs Jones,' said the teacher. 'Come along, I'll show you to your classes. You're in Junior One, Miss Sykes' class,' says Mrs Jones. She then turns to Grahame. 'And you boy are in Junior Two, just through that door.' Mrs Jones takes me to my class.
'Now this is Lorraine,' says Miss Sykes, 'she's come to join our class.'
The kids all stare at me and I feel a bit strange.
My stomach aches; I don't like been the new girl.
'Sit down dear' says Miss Sykes, pointing to a seat at the front of the room.

I look around the classroom. It's not as big as the classroom at my last school and it seems very strange to be sitting next to a boy.
The boy's name is Alan. He has ginger hair and a face full of freckles. He doesn't talk to me very much. Opposite me sits a tall

girl with long brown plaits. She smiles at me. She has got a nice friendly face and I hope she is going to be my friend.

'We're going across to the field this morning to play rounders with Class Three, so I want you all to line up against the door' says Miss Sykes.

The school field is enormous, much bigger than the one at my last school, in fact that one just looked like a large patch of grass in comparison to this one.
Two girls are sitting making daisy chains. I walk over to them. One of the girls is the girl that sits near me in the class. The other one has long blonde hair and blue eyes. She smiles at me.
'Hello,' I say, remembering to use a posh voice.
The blond haired girl looks at me and smiles.
'Hiya,' she says.
'Oh,' I say, surprised because the girl didn't sound at all posh, 'Oh erm hiya.'
The two girls look at each other and start laughing.
'What's your name?' says the blonde girl.
'Lorraine, Lorraine Tranmer.'
I saw you moving in; you live down the lane, don't you?'
'Yes, and it's lovely.'
'I live down the lane. Our bungalow isn't far from yours.'
I turn to the other girl.
'Do you live down the lane?' I ask.
'No, I live down George Street.'
'What are your names?'
'I'm Claire,' says the blonde girl
'And I'm Pat,' says her friend.
At that moment the whistle is blown.
'See you after school, wait for me outside my class' says Claire.
'She's in Junior Three,' says Pat as we join the other kids on the field. 'In 'Fanny Adams' class.'
I walk along smiling to myself, for I had made two friends already and they weren't at all posh, in fact there were very nice, so Dianne had been wrong.

Chapter 16

'Do you know what Fuck means?' says Claire on the way home from school.

'Well I know it's a real bad word, me Mam would kill me if she heard me saying that.'

'Yes but do you know what it means?'

'Of course I do,' I say.

'Well what does it mean then?'

'It means go away; it's just a naughty way of telling someone to get lost, you tell them to fuck off," I say in a whisper.

'It means something else as well,' says Claire

'Oh well, what does it mean?' I say, feeling a bit fed up.

'Well, do you know where babies come from?'

'Yes, the nurse brings them in her bag.'

Claire throws her head back and laughs. Her long blonde hair glistens in the sunlight.

'They grow in the woman's stomach,' she says. 'And do you know how they get there?'

'No, no I don't,' I say, feeling a bit stupid.

'Well,' says Claire, her eyes widening, 'the man does rude things to the woman.'

'Oh, what things?'

'Well the man puts his thingy on the woman's stomach and her 'you know', and his seed goes inside her and it makes a baby.'

'Don't lie, my Mam and Dad would never do that!'

'They have,' says Claire tossing her head back. 'How do you think you were born?

The man likes it but I don't think the woman likes it very much.'

'A man did that to me once,' I say, ' but I never grew a baby.'

Claire looks shocked. 'Did you tell your Mam?' she asks.

'Yes, I did.'

'Well what did the coppers say?'

'Me Mam never told the coppers.'

'You mean he did that to you and no one did anything?'

I shrug my shoulders. 'Shall we go picking flowers tonight?' I say.

'But my Mam would have gone to the coppers.' says Claire. 'She wouldn't let anyone do things like that to me.'

'There're some nice flowers growing by drain bank,' I say.

'I don't think anyone cares about you,' says Claire, 'or they

wouldn't have let him get away with it.'
'Yes they do!' I say as I run off.

I slam into our home.
'What on earth's the matter with you?' says my Mam, looking at my
tear stained face.
'Nothing,' I reply sulkily.
"There must be something the matter; I can see you've been crying.'
'Oh, I fell and banged me arm,' I lie as I go into my bedroom.
'Let me have a look, it it could be broken or something.'
I'm all right, it doesn't hurt now,' I mutter before slamming my
bedroom door.
Once inside my bedroom I throw myself on to the bed. Claire's
words are going round and round in my head: *no one care about*
you, no one cares about you.
Putting the cover over my head I cry myself to sleep.
I wake up about an hour later.
'Your tea's ready' I hear my Mam shout.
'I don't want any,' I shout back, 'I'm not hungry.'
I sit up in bed, lost in thought.
I think about what happened to me and try to sort out in my mind
why my Mam didn't tell the police about what Uncle Ralph had
done. She must care about me I reason with myself; she's my Mam.
But why wasn't anything done? Surely they didn't think I would
just forget it had ever happened?
'What's wrong with you? Don't you feel very well?' says my Mam
coming to my room.
'Why don't you want any tea?'
'I'm just not hungry'
'Has something happened at school, something that has upset you?'
I shake my head.
'No I just want to be on my own for a little bit.'
'But why Lorraine? Tell me what's wrong.'
I want to ask me Mam if she cares about me and tell her that she
should have told the police about Uncle Ralph. But my throat has
got a big lump in it and my mouth feels dry and parched. All I can
do is shake my head.
'Stop playing with your food and eat it up,' says my dad.
I ignore him and continue pushing the food round my plate.
'Oh Lorraine, you haven't eaten a blooming thing.' My Mam looks
at me crossly.

'I went to a lot of trouble to get your tea ready so get it eaten,' she says.

Grahame holds his fork in the air, 'I'll eat hers if she doesn't want it,' he says.

'You'll do nowt of the sort,' says me dad, 'now Lorraine, get the bugger eaten or you're not going out to play.'

'I don't wanna play out,' I say, 'and I'm not going to eat it. You can't force me so get lost.'

My dad glares at me sternly. 'Well in that case you can get to bloody bed,' he snaps.

I get up and flounce to my bedroom door. 'See if I care,' I say boldly.

'Get to bed now!' says my dad.

I shrug my shoulders and once again slam the bedroom door behind me.

Chapter 17

'Come on Lorraine get up it's time you got ready for school.'
'I'm not going,' I say sullenly.
'What's wrong?' says my Mam.
'Just not going,' I say.
'But you like school,'
'No I don't, it's horrible.'
'Come on, get out of that bed, there's nowt wrong with you. I think you're just being lazy this morning. Come and have something to eat. You must be hungry, you never ate a thing for your tea.'
Hesitantly I get out of bed. I don't want to go to school. I'm worried Claire has told everyone what I said to her about that Uncle Ralph, and what if they all think that my Mam and Dad don't care about me?

'Hurry up, you're going to be late,' says my Mam looking at the clock.
I slowly dress.
'Bye then love, see you after school,' says my Mam giving me a kiss.
I turn away and walk out of the door.

Claire is waiting for me at the gate.
'You all right?' she says.
I nod my head.
'Come on then, let's get moving.'
We walk down the lane. I drag my feet.
'What's wrong?' asks Claire.
'Nowt,' I mumble.
'Is it about what we talked about yesterday about when you know, that happened to you?'
I shrug my shoulders. 'You won't tell anyone will you?' I ask in a small voice.
'No, I promise,' says Claire.
'Good.'
'You're my bestest friend now,' says Claire, cuddling me.

We arrive at the school but despite what Claire has said I am still worrying in case she does tell anyone.

'Lorraine, you haven't written down one single word!' says the teacher as she collects up the papers from the spelling test. 'You haven't even bothered to write your name at the top.'

I bite down hard on my bottom lip whilst a boy sneers at me.

'Why haven't you written anything? I know you are capable of doing it.'

There is a silence.

The boy looks on smugly and I can feel everyone staring at me.

'Well?' said the teacher, 'I'm waiting. Why haven't you done your spellings?'

'Didn't wanna,' I mutter.

'I beg your pardon?'

I lower my head, unable to think straight. I could have done the spellings, they were easy, but I just couldn't seem to get anything down on the paper as my head was all full up with jumbled thoughts and worries. All I managed to do during the test was stare down at the blank square of paper before me.

'You can stay in all playtime,' said the teacher crossly.

The boy sniggers at me and I put my tongue out at him.

'You insolent child!' says the teacher, pulling me out of my seat.

I feel my cheeks flame as the teacher slaps the backs of my legs in front of the whole class. The tears well up in my eyes but I blink them back as the boy smirks and watches me intently.

'You will sit there and write out twenty times 'I MUST NOT BE RUDE AND DISOBEDIENT, ' says my teacher, slamming a piece of paper and a blunt stubby pencil down in front of me.

I sit at my desk. The sun shines through the window and I can hear the other kids playing happily outside in the playground.

'Well get on with it then.' My teacher glares at me from behind her desk.

I slowly pick up the pen. My stomach aching, I begin to write.

After what seems like hours I hear the ringing of the school bell.

The teachers looks up from her desk. 'Well, have you finished?' she says.

She glides across to my desk and picks up the paper.

'I said twenty times!' she snaps, 'you have only written eight lines and...' says my teacher as though I had committed the most unforgivable sin, 'you have spelt disobedient wrong. Perhaps if you had done your spelling test you would have spelt it correctly.'

The other kids enter the classroom and return to their seats.

'You can come out and sit at the front of the class,' says my teacher, 'then I can keep my eye on you.'

The day passes slowly until at long last it is time to go home.

'You had better behave yourself tomorrow,' says the teacher as I walk towards the door, 'because if you don't I will send you straight to see the headmaster and you won't get way with things quite so easily then.'

I walk out of the classroom and step onto the playground.

'Class's dunce, class's dunce,' taunts the boy who had been sniggering at me. 'Can't even spell, class's dunce, class's dunce!

The boy dances round me. I want to push him out of the way. I'm so mad that I want to just hit him and hit him and not stop.

Claire runs over to me. 'Take no notice of him, he's just bloody stupid,' she says.

Ignoring the boy Claire links her arm in mine and we walk away.

Claire is not in my class so she doesn't know anything about what had happened in school that morning. When I tell her her eyes widen like saucers, 'You'd better not get sent to Jonesl,' she says, 'because my big brother told me that he has a cane.'

'I'm not bothered,' I mutter, shrugging my shoulders.

We walk on in silence until we reach the top of our lane.

'What's wrong?' asks Claire, 'you're very quiet.'

'Oh nowt really.'

We wander down the lane.

'Is it about what happened to you? You know, when you were little.'

I give an annoyed sigh.

'Well don't worry about it, 'cos you know you can talk to me about 'owt', don't you?'

I smile, feeling a bit better. I had got a friend and she was the best friend in the whole world and she cared about me.

'What are you doing after tea, you playing out? We could go for a walk down the drain bank or down the tracks.'

I nod my head eagerly. We reach Claire's bungalow. It's painted green and has the name ROSEDENE printed in big letters just above one of the windows.

'Had a good day?' asks my Mam as I walk in.

'All right,' I mutter.

'I hope you're in a better mood then you were this morning.'

'What's for tea Mam?' asks Grahame.

My Mam sighs. 'Stewed bugs and onions,' she says.

'No 'yike onions,' says little Michael.

I look across at Michael and smile. He's lovely is our little Michael, he makes me laugh.

He's two now and my Mam says he can talk very well for his age. When you ask him his name he points to himself and says in a very important voice 'De Marple.' His name for me is Naney as he can't say Lorraine. It's great watching a baby grow, I can't believe he was once that tiny little scrap that lay in that blue carry cot just one hour old.

I sometimes take him for walks in his tansad and show him off to my friends.

I'm so proud of my little brother, he's funny and very clever, he can count to seven and knows lots of nursery rhymes.

I can't wait for school to break up for the long summer holidays, then I will be able to play out all day and forget about everything.

Chapter 18

'Those blooming chickens have knocked my milk over again,' says my Mam, walking into the house.

Mr Mitchel's chickens were always coming onto our land.

'That's the third time they've done that this week.' My Mam has a worried look on her face. 'What with your Father on strike and everything I'm having trouble making ends meet as it is,' she went on, almost to herself. Sighing, my Mam peers into our small food cupboard and then counts the change in her purse. 'Well, it looks like it will have to be stew for dinner,' she says.

'Not again,' mutters Grahame. 'There's no meat left in it, just bones, and we always have meat on a Sunday.'

'Well it's either that or starve,' says my Mam. She then turns to my dad. 'I'll be glad when you are back at work Doug,' she says, 'I can hardly cope.'

'Well we would be daft going back now Jean love, it's better that we stick to our guns.' My dad sighs and makes himself scarce.

'I'm hungry now,' says Grahame as he spreads jam onto his bread.

If there isn't much else in the food cupboard there are plenty of jars full of bramble jam. My Mam makes it, it tastes lovely, but after a while you get a bit sick of the taste of brambles.

'I think I'll go fishing in the drain,' says Grahame.

Grahame often goes fishing in the drain. He catches eels and my dad cooks them in milk.

I turned my nose up at them at first.

'I'm not eating those slimy looking things,' I said.

'Just try them,' said my dad, 'They're a delicacy in London you know; people pay a fortune for them.'

My dad then pushed a small forkful into my mouth and to my surprise I found they tasted very nice.

'Can I come fishing with you Grahame?' I ask

'No,' says Grahame, 'you stay and play with your stupid dolls. Fishing is for boys.'

'I don't play with dolls any more, so there' I say.

'Well, you're still not coming with me.'

I poke my tongue out at my brother and he clouts me across my head.

'Mam Mam! He hit me!' I yell.

'Will you two stop falling out? I just can't cope what with your dad on strike and everything.'

At that moment my dad walks back into the house. He has a chicken feather stuck to his cheek. 'Dinner's in the shed Jean love,' is all he says before sitting down with his paper.

Some time later instead of the stew we have chicken.

'This tastes lovely,' I say.

'Compliments of Mr Mitchel' laughs Grahame.

'What do you mean?' I ask

'Well a couple of chickens wondered into our shed and my dad necked the buggers,' says Grahame proudly.

'Well that will pay for all the bottles of milk they have knocked over,' says my Mam.

My dad turns to me. 'Come on, eat your dinner love.'

Chapter 19

'Where do you live?' ask the two girls in the playground.
'Down the lane,' I say with a smile.
'The lane?'
'What lane?'
She means down Bonds Street,' says a boy with a sneer.
'Bonds street.'
'So you live on Bonds estate.' The two girls look at each other and laugh.
'My mother says it's a shanty town.'
'Well my mother won't even let me go down there.'
'Why?' I ask. 'It's a lovely place.'
'Because all the scruffy people and the gippos live down there and my dad says that Bonds estate is the slum of Hedon.'
'Go away,' I say, wanting to burst into tears. 'It's nice down the lane. You're just being stupid.'
'Do you want a fight?' says the biggest girl.
I try to walk away.
'I'm going to get you after school tonight' she hisses.
'Take no notice of them two,' says Claire as she walks up to me, 'they're just snobs.'

'You've hardly done any of those sums I set you,' says the teacher as she collects up our sum books. 'Make sure you try harder tomorrow.'
I look at the clock on the wall. It's nearly home time, the time I have been dreading.
We all sing 'Now the day is over', and then leave the classroom.

As I leave the playground I feel a hand grab my shoulder. I turn around and I'm faced with the girl who had threatened me.
'I'm going to kick your flipping head in,' she snarls, balling her hand into a tight fist.
I step back. Her fists rain down on my face. By this time a crowd has gathered. They are all shouting and spurring the girl on. Not knowing what to do I pull the girl's hair and grab hold off her face with my hands. The girl lets out a scream but I keep hold of her face. Suddenly a teacher breaks us up. I look at the girl; her cheek is streaming with blood from where my nails have dug into her cheek.

'Cat fighter,' hisses one of her friends as I'm frogmarched back into the school.

'We will deal with you in the morning,' says the headmaster. ' We don't have fighting like that in this school.'
With trembling legs I walk out of the headmaster's office.

'I wonder what made her do such a thing,' I hear the teacher say.
'Well you can't expect anything else' mutters another, 'she is from the back streets.'

Claire pats my back as we walk home. 'Well done!' she says. 'She's had it coming has that one, not many people dare stand up to her.'
'I didn't mean it,' I say 'I didn't mean to make her bleed.'
'Well, I'm glad you did' laughs Claire.
We walk on in silence.
Grahame is standing at the top of the lane. 'Is it true,' he asks, 'about you having a fight with that horrible lass?'
'Yeah, and you should have seen her, she didn't half give her what for' says Claire.
Grahame smiles. 'I'm glad,' he says, 'she's a right stuck up bitch if ever there was one.'
We walk into the house. The television is on and Michael is sitting engrossed in The Clangers.
'Look at the state of you,' says my Mam, taking in my dishevelled appearance.
'She's been in a fight,' says Grahame proudly.
'What on earth have you been fighting about?' My Mam shakes her head, giving me an icy stare.
'Well it was this lass, she started it,' I stammer, 'sh...she said nasty things about our lane and then when I was coming out of school she hit me real hard.'
My mother's face softened. 'And so you hit her back?' she says, nodding her head.
'Yes she did, and she won the fight,' laughs Grahame.
'Well, you did right hitting her back, you have to stick up for yourself' says my Mam.

By the time I reach school the next day word had got around about the fight.
'You're a cat fighter, you pull hair and scratch,' said a boy in my

class.

Not many of the kids are very friendly towards me and some of them jeer behind my back, 'Cat fighter, cat fighter.'

'Well, she's only little,' says Claire, coming to my defence, 'you can't expect her to punch very well with her tiny hands.'

I enter my classroom and just as I'm sitting down at my desk the headmaster walks through the door. He fixes me with a stony stare whilst he speaks to our teacher.

The headmaster leaves the class and my teacher tells me to go and wait outside the headmaster's office.

I'm left waiting outside the office for some time before the headmaster finally calls my name. With legs like jelly I enter his office and stand facing the headmaster who is sitting behind a large desk.

The headmaster glares at me. 'Why did you attack Debbie?' he says.

I look down at the floor.

'Stand up straight girl, and tell me why you attacked Debbie.'

'I didn't m...mean it,' I stutter, 'she hit me f...first.'

'It makes no difference!' shouts the headmaster, 'you must never fight. We don't have fighting in this school you know.'

'B...ut bu...t she hit me.'

'Let me look at your nails,' says the headmaster, ignoring me.

He looks at my rather long nails and tuts to himself.

'I want you to see Mrs Harris and get them cut immediately. They're far too long and grubby.

'But before you go I want you to know that we don't tolerate fighting in this school and for attacking Debbie you will stay in every day at playtime for two whole weeks, and,' the head raises his hand and points to a thin bamboo cane in the corner, 'if you do this again you will be punished more severely.'

I return to my classroom.

'You can sit at the front of the class,' said the teacher, 'so that I can see what you're doing.'

That morning whilst the other kids did painting I was given a sheet of hard sums to do. When the kids go out to play I'm left inside with just the teacher scowling at me from her desk.

Chapter 20

'What's wrong with you,' says my Mam, 'You've hardly said a word all teatime.'

'She's been in trouble with old Jones for hitting that lass,' says Grahame.

'But she hit her in self defence,' says my Mam, turning to my dad.

'It's not our Lorraine that should be in bother, it's the other one.' My Mam shakes her head. 'I'm not having it Doug,' she says, 'I'll be going to that school first thing in the morning.

'My Mam does care about me,' I say to Claire as we walk down the drain bank.

'She can't do,' says Claire, 'or else she would have-'

'She does! She's going to school in the morning about old Jones telling me off an...and she says it wasn't my fault' I say, all in in a rush.

Claire sighs and shakes her head.

I look up at her confused, wanting her to agree with me, but she just shrugs her shoulders and doesn't say anything.

'Look, there's a water rat in there,' I say, pointing to the murky water in the drain.

But Claire doesn't even follow my gaze and just carries on walking. We reach our bungalow.

'See you then,' says Claire as she stops at our gate.

'But I'm not going in yet, can't we go climbing trees?'

'I'm off to me Grans.'

Claire walks on.

'See you then,' I say. Claire doesn't say anything, she just walks off leaving me standing at my gate.

I watch as she disappears from my sight, not knowing what to believe or what to think. I try hard to reason with myself that yes, Mam and Dad do care about me, Claire had been wrong. However, questions still linger in the back of my mind. Questions I feel are too difficult to ask. So I decide to just leave them where they are and try not to think about them too much.

Chapter 21

Me Mam's getting a fat belly again because she has a baby growing inside it. She told me last night and I'm very excited. It's due to be born in September when we all go back to school after the six week holiday. I can't wait for my new sister or brother to be born.

I look at my Mam's belly as she sits in her chair and try to imagine how it must feel to be a little baby squashed up tight in a small place, waiting to be born.
I'd seen pictures like this in the MIND ALIVE Magazine my dad buys.

I sit and watch as she knits, expertly twisting and turning the white wool over the metal pointed needles.
A slow smile spreads over her face and for some reason I just want to hug her. But I don't, I just sit watching her knit whilst listening to the comfortable click click click of the needles.
Sensing my gaze my Mam smiles. 'It'll be lovely when the new baby's born,' she says. 'You were a lovely baby you know, Lorraine.'
'Was I good?'
'You were,' says my Mam, 'and you still are a good lass.' My Mam sighs 'I hope you are going to help me look after the new baby.'.
'Of course I will Mam.'
'Oh, I am glad. Babies are lovely but they're a lot of hard work.'
My Mam pats her smock top. 'But I suppose they're worth it,' she says, almost to herself.
'What's that you're knitting Mam?'
'Just a little matinee jacket for the new baby.' My Mam reaches in her knitting bag and fetches out a tiny pair of booties. 'These are to go with it,' she says.
'Oh Mam, aren't they nice?'
My Mam pats her belly again. 'Well I'll have to get on with me knitting. I've only about three weeks to go before it's born.'
'I hope it's a lad,' says Grahame.
'But I want a little sister.'
'Well it's going to be a lad, I just know it is, so there' says Grahame.
'We'll just have to wait and see,' says my Mam.
My Mam carries on with her knitting and there is a comfortable silence in the small room. I pick up the latest copy of the MIND

ALIVE which is lying on the couch and flick through the pages. I stop at the centre page and my heart goes into my mouth, for there is a picture of a women giving birth to a baby. Her face is screwed up in pain and there is a lot of blood. The baby is very ugly and wrinkled. My heart beating fast, I quickly close the magazine, but the vision of the woman's face and the ugly baby is still in my mind. Suddenly I don't care any more; I'm not bothered if the baby is a little boy as long as my Mam's all right and the baby isn't as ugly and bloody as the one in the MIND ALIVE.

My Mam stops her knitting. 'I think it's time you two went to bed,' she says.

'But Mam, it's the six weeks holiday,' protests Grahame.

My Mam looks at the clock. 'Well you can have ten more minutes and then it's bedtime.'

'I'm off fishing in the drain tomorrow,' says Grahame. 'There's nowt much in there but a few boot laces but the cat likes 'em.'

I laugh as I remember that the last time Grahame had been fishing in the drain Lydia our cat had waited on the drain bank. Then when Grahame reeled in an eel she suddenly pounced onto the fishing line. The line swung across the drain with the cat attached to it like grim death.

Grahame pats the cat on the head. 'You like fishing, don't you Lyd?' he says.

My Mam lays her knitting down on her knee and inspects the stitches.

'Well, that's coming on nice,' she says.

I look at her and smile. She smiles back. I walk up to her and kiss her cheek.

'Night night Mam, I'll see you in morning.'

Suddenly my Mam jumps. She puts my hand on her smock top.

'Can you feel it? That's the baby kicking.'

I feel the ripple on my Mams smock top, then a little bump.

'That will be a little foot,' says me Mam.

A sudden surge of panic runs through me as I remember the picture I'd seen in the MIND ALIVE.

'Do you feel all right Mam?' I ask.

'Of course I do love,' says my Mam, 'women have babies every day. Now off you get to bed.'

Chapter 22

September the ninth 1967

My Mam had got so fat she could hardly walk and I could tell she's in pain as she had been holding her side all day. She hadn't eaten her tea either. We sit and watch the television but I can't concentrate on the programme as I'm worried about my Mam.

My dad puts our Michael to bed and then turns to me and our Grahame.

'Come on you two,' he says, 'get yourselves to bed.'

'But Dad, it's only early,' says Grahame.'

My dad points to our bedroom door. 'Bed!' he shouts, 'right now, your Mam isn't very well.'

Reluctantly we go to bed.

****

I lie there in the dark. It's getting late; Grahame had fallen sleep ages ago but I can't. I know that something isn't right.

Suddenly I hear the front door open and then my Auntie's voice.

Are you all right lass? Is the ambulance on its way?'

'Yes,' says my Mam, in between breaths. 'Doug went to Mrs Ward's and rang one up.'

'How often are you getting them?'

'The pains?'

'Aye.'

'Oh it's only early days yet, about every half an hour. It was Doug that insisted on getting the ambulance out.'

'Well he did right.' says Auntie. 'You can't be too careful.'

I hear my Mam groan and tears well up in my eyes.

'Take it easy love,' says Auntie.

Suddenly after what seems like ages I hear the front door open again.

'The ambulance is waiting' says a man's voice.

My Mam groans again.

'Just relax love, we'll have you there as quick as we can.'

'Have you got your case?' says my Auntie.

'Aye, everything's ready,' says my Mam.

'See you soon then love.'

'It will be all over next time I see you. Bye Auntie, thanks for looking after the bairns.'

I heard my Mam and dad and the ambulance man leave the house and for some reason I put the covers over my head. Tears fell down my face and I prayed to God that my Mam will be all right. 'Dear God,' I mutter quietly, 'I know I never say my prayers but I promise I will say them every night if you see that me Mam is all right.

I don't even care if the new baby is ugly, please look after me Mam. Amen.'

I lay there for hours. My stomach ached and my mouth felt dry. Finally my eyelids started pricking and I felt myself drifting to sleep.

'You've got a new baby brother!' shouts my dad. I wake up and rub the sleep from my eyes. My dad has a big smile on his face and he seems really happy.

Grahame jumps up and down on the bed. 'I knew we would get another little brother!' he whoops, 'I just knew it.'

'He's a big lad,' says my dad. 'Eight pound fourteen ounces.'

'And me Mam,' I say, 'is she all right?'

'She's fine love,' says my dad.

My dad leaves our bedroom and I join in, jumping up and down on my bed with excitement, not at all bothered that the baby isn't a girl.

'Shall we make the new baby a little toy?' says Grahame when we'd settled down.

'Well, what can we make?'

'We can make a sort of gonk.'

'But we haven't got any material,' I say.

Grahame then picks up one of his grey socks off the floor. 'Well we could use this,' he says.

'What can we do with that?'

We could just cut the top off, stuff it to make a head then make some feet with what we've cut off.'

I agreed that this was a good idea so we set to work on making the gonk.

'I'll stuff it, cut the feet out and you can sew it up 'cos sewing is for lasses,' says Grahme, taking handfuls of spongy stuffing from his pillow.

When Grahame had finished I then set about the task of sewing it up. I used buttons for the gonks eyes and using red embroidery thread which my Gran had given me I stitched on a nose and a big smiley mouth.

'That looks great,' says Grahame, 'the baby will love it.'

That night my dad was going to see my Mam in hospital.

'Wev'e made the baby a gonk' I say. Grahame then proudly shows my dad the toy.

My dad has a big smile spread all over his face. 'That's lovely,' he says, 'I'll take it to him tonight.'

'The new baby loves the toy,' says my dad as he walks into the house after visiting my Mam.

'How's me Mam?' I ask

'Oh she's a bit tired but apart from that she's fine.'

'When is she coming home?' asks Grahame.

'In about nine days.'

Dad, why couldn't she have had the baby in her own bed? Why did she have to go into hospital?' I ask.

'On account of the toilet,' says my dad, 'but don't worry, your Mam's fine.'

'The toilet?'

'Aye,' says my dad. 'It's an earth toilet, not a flush one. The nurse didn't think it was quite right.'

'I see.'

'But lots of babies was born down this lane when I was a lad and they never ailed nowt, a bit bloody stupid as far as I can see. But still, your Mam needs her rest so I suppose hospital's the best place for her.'

'I can't wait to see the new baby and I'm missing me Mam already,' I say.

'Well she'll be home soon,' says my dad. 'You'll see her then.'

The six weeks holiday have come to an end and today is the start of the new school term.

I put my coat on and walk up our long path. Grahame has already set off because he starts South Holderness today and he has to walk all the way to Preston which is about two miles away from the bottom of our lane. He looked so different in his new school uniform with the grey blazer, grey trousers, shirt and tie. My Mam says it cost a lot of money and he has to get changed the moment he comes home from school. But I don't think Grahame's bothered about that fact at all. My friend Claire is also starting big school today. I feel a bit sad because it will seem very strange in the playground without her.

As I walk through the school gates I see my friend Pat.
'Iv'e got a new baby brother,' I say, smiling. 'He was born early this morning.'
'Thought you wanted a sister,' says Pat, unimpressed.
'I did, but I'm not bothered now.'

'What his name then?' says Pat.
'Whose name?'
'The new baby's.'
'I don't know, we haven't thought of one yet.'

'I hate first days,' says Pat.
'So do I.'
'Whose class are you gonna be in?'
'Fanny Adam's,' I sigh.
'Poor you,' says Pat, 'she's horrible.'
I feel a bit sad because we won't be in the same class any more as Pat is going in Mr Felix's class. We enter the playground and the school bell is rung. Our names are called out and we all line up outside our new classrooms.
'See you at playtime,' says Pat.

Chapter 23

'What are we going to call him then?' says my Mam as we gaze at our new baby brother.

'Baby,' says little Michael.

We all look at Michael and laugh.

'We can't just call him baby,' I say.

My Mam holds the baby on her knee with a look of contentment on her face. 'I like the name Ivan,' says my Mam.

'Yes that's a good name Jean,' agrees my dad.

Grahame shakes his head. 'No, I don't like it' he says.

'Why not?' asks my Mam.

'Well it's a bit sort of sissy.'

'I hate it,' I say, 'it's a horrible name.'

'But I think it suits him,' says my Mam.

I look at my baby brother and decide that he doesn't look at all like an Ivan.

'I don't like the name, I think it's …'

'Look, if your Mam likes it then that's what we call him,' interrupts my dad crossly.

'No,' says my Mam, 'we must all decide what to call him.'

'I love the name David,' I say.

'Well what about Chris?' says Grahame.

'Ther're both nice names,' smiles my Mam looking down at our little brother.

'How about if we call him David Christopher.'

We all nod our heads and so the new baby is now called David.

I'm glad; David's a lot nicer name than Ivan.

****

The house is quiet. My dad and our Grahame have gone fishing. My Mam sits by the fire with David on her knee. She looks up at me and smiles.

'Do you want to hold your new baby brother?' she asks.

I nod my head eagerly.

Me Mam places a large cushion on my side. 'Sit back,' she says. She then place's David in my arms. I gaze down into David's face. He is wide awake and his big blue eyes look into mine. His tiny hand is rolled into a little fist which he keeps putting to his mouth.

'He's ready for a feed,' says my Mam, 'do you want to give him his bottle?'

Although a little nervous I nod my head eagerly. My Mam disappears into the kitchen.

'Won't be long,' she says.

David starts to cry a little. He sounds like a little kitten. I hold him closer to me. He smells lovely a sort of warm sweet smell. I stroke his soft wisps of dark hair and then trace my finger lightly on his face. His skin is so soft and for some reason a lump forms in my throat.

Me Mam returns from the kitchen with a titty bottle filled with milk. She hands it to me.

'Now hold the bottle up,' she says as I put the teat into David's searching mouth.

'Don't let him swallow wind or he will get colic.' My Mam places the cushion under my arm. I sit there watching as David slowly sucks from the bottle. He looks up at me. His eyes never leave my face. He look so trusting.

'You're doing real well Lorraine,' smiles my Mam.

'You will make a good little mother one day; it seems to come naturally to you.'

I hold my little brother closer and at that moment I feel a strong wave of protectiveness towards him.

'Now take the bottle out and pat his back,' says my Mam. 'That will help get his wind up.'

David cries when I take the rubber teat from out of his mouth. I sit him up and gently pat his back.

'No, like this,' says my Mam. She takes David out of my arms and rubs his back harder. Very soon David gives a little burp. 'That's it, clever boy,' she says to him as she puts the teat back into his mouth. I watch as David finishes his feed.

Sleepy now, David lies in her arms. A thin dribble of milk covers his chin. My Mam kisses him lightly on the forehead and carefully places him in the wooden rocking cradle. David settles down contentedly and very soon he is fast asleep.

'Isn't he lovely Mam?' I say, looking down at my little brother.

'He is,' says my Mam, smiling.

At that moment our little Michael toddles into the room. He's been playing outside in the garden. He is wearing his little cowboy outfit and has a huge smile on his little freckled face. His eyes are lit up and full of mischief. My heart melts when I look at him, so I pick him up and sit him on my knee.

'Aren't we lucky Mam,' I say.

'We are that,' says my Mam. 'We might not have a lot of money but we are really lucky.'

'I can't wait to have a baby of my own' I say, almost to myself.

My Mam looks at me quizzically. 'What was that you said Lorrraine?' she says.

'Oh nothing Mam,' I mutter.

******

The weeks and months flew past and before I knew it David had cut his first tooth and had taken his first stumbling step. Life went by in a haze of long walks, fishing, making dens and tree climbing. And then when the colder weather came we settled down to dark nights as we waited for winter to arrive. When the snow came the lane was transformed into a magical place. Much to the kids' delight the council hardly ever put any grit down on the lane, making it a haven for kids but treacherous for the old people.

Most of my time was spent slipping and sliding down the hill at the corner near Shan's Land and on the frozen water logged fields and ponds.

However, when the thaw arrived the lane was messy and grey sludge splattered up your socks as you walked, or seeped through the holes in your Wellington boots.

The potholes were full of dirty water which were often difficult to avoid as you walked along, and by the time I'd got to school my once white socks were filthy.

Everyone welcomed the spring when it came to the lane and then when the summer came and winter was long forgotten, my Mam would hardly ever see us.

I'll never forget the summer Pat and a friend called Pete and I went to Burstwick ski pit.

Burstwick was about four miles away and Pete was the only one with a bike. So I walked along the road whilst Pete gave Pat a crossbar ride on his bike. Then he dropped her off and came back for me. Eventually we all arrived at the ski pit. It was a hot day and the moment we got there we took off our shoes and socks and began to paddle at the edge of the water. Pete was wearing his shorts. 'I'm going to swim all the way round,' he said.

"Be careful Pete, my dad told me that the pit has no bottom, just sinking gravel.'

'I'll be all right, I'm a good swimmer.'

I hardly dared watch as Pete swam bravely around the ski pit.

"What if he drowns?' I said to Pat.

Pat laughed. 'He won't,' she said. 'Don't be daft.' She then looks at me closely.

'You like Pete, don't you?' she says.

I nod my head.

'Well he's my big sister's boyfriend,' she said.

"I know,' I reply quietly, 'he's too old for me anyway.'

The day ended all too quickly and we made our way home.

Pat was right, I did like Pete, in fact he was the first boy I'd ever really liked, he was funny and nice and he made me laugh.

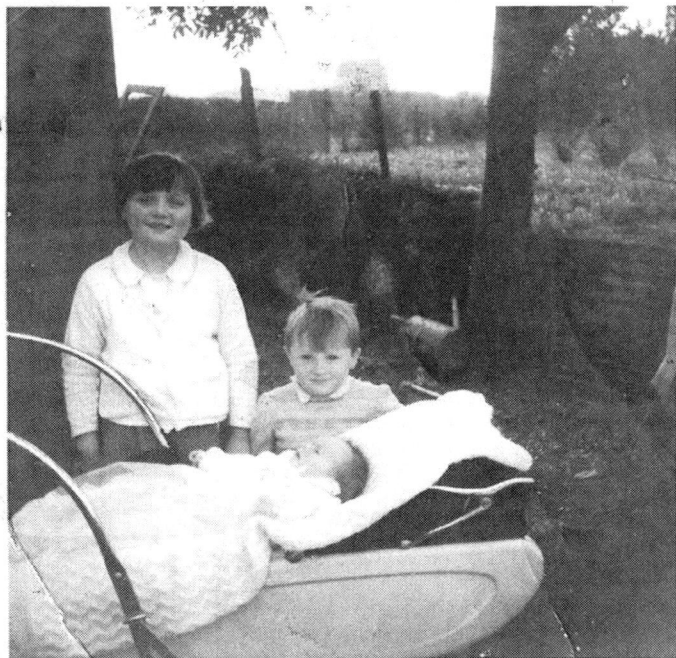

The new baby, David Christopher, our little Michael and me down
Bonds Street, Hedon, summer 1967.

Chapter 24

You're going on a little holiday,' says my Mam.
'Where to?' asks Grahame.
'Withernsea, for a whole week,' says my Mam.
'When are we going?' I ask.
'In a week's time but the thing is,' says my Mam, 'only you and Grahame are going.'
'What? Do you mean we're going away without you?'
'That's right love. You are going to stay with a nice family, you see,' went on my Mam. 'What with your dad losing his job and everything we haven't been able to afford a holiday in a long time, so a nice couple have said that they will let you and Grahame stay with them in Withernsea.'
Grahame and I look at each other.
'Just think,' says my Mam, 'you'll be able to go on the beach every day and I'll give you some money for the amusements. It will be a little break for me as well,' says my Mam, 'what with the baby and everything. You know I could do with a little rest.'
'Oh that will be smashing Mam,' I say. 'I love the seaside.'
Grahame didn't look too impressed with the idea. 'But Mam,' he protested, 'it's the last week of our six weeks so when we get back we will be going back to school. I think I would rather stay here down the lane than go to Withernsea.'
'Don't be daft' says my Mam. 'It will be a nice change for you, you will be able to go swimming in the sea, I thought you liked swimming.'
Grahame considers the prospect for a short while, then he cheers up,
Over the next few days Grahame and I began to look forward to our holiday.

The day of the holiday arrives with the sun shining high in the sky.
My Mam, Grahame and myself make our way down the lane. We are on our way to meet Mrs Smith, the lady who we were going to stay with.
'Now I want you both to be good,' says my Mam as we walk along, 'and no falling out.'

We enter the Welfare Office. A grey haired lady sitting behind a desk smiles at us.

'So you're Grahame and Lorraine,' she says. She looks closely at us. 'I hear you are going on a little holiday; what lucky children you are,' she beams. I didn't like the woman very much; it was the way she spoke to us like we were five year olds and not eleven and twelve.

Presently a fat fair haired woman bustles through the door. She is wearing a faded dress with large flowers on it and a blue cardigan.

'Ah, Mrs Smith,' smiles the woman behind the desk. 'Now this is Grahame and Lorraine,' she says.

'I hope you haven't been waiting long.' Mrs Smith smiles at me, while the woman behind the desk speaks quietly to my Mam.

My Mam then told us both to be good, gave us both a kiss and left the room.

'Come along then kids,' says Mrs Smith.

We follow Mrs Smith down the street and stop where a grey car is parked. A fat dumpy man is sitting behind the steering wheel.

Mrs Smith opens the car door. 'Hop in then kids,' she says.

Grahame climbs into the car but I hesitate. For some reason I just want to run and go back home with my Mam.

'Come on dear,' says Mrs Smith.

Holding back my tears I get into the car and sit on the back seat with Grahame.

The car has a musky smoky sort of smell. The man behind the steering wheel turns around and faces me.

'We'll soon be there kids,' he says. 'They're all waiting for you.'

The car speeds along. I look out of the window. A lump forms in my throat as we leave Hedon behind.

After what seems like ages I see a sign which says: WITHERNSEA WELCOMES YOU.

'Nearly there kids,' says Mrs Smith.

Mr Smith turns down a street with lots of big houses on one side of the road and smaller ones on the other side. Mr Smith stops the car outside one of the big houses. He comes around to our door and opens it wide.

'Hop out kids,' he says.

We get out of the car and follow Mr and Mrs Smith down the path. Mr Smith opens the door. I hesitate on the step. Mrs Smith takes my hand and leads me into the hallway. 'Come and meet everyone,' she says.

We walk into a room at the end of the hallway. There seem to be kids everywhere.

The room smells strongly of babies' dirty nappies and bad cabbage. A girl of about my age walks up to me. 'Hiya,' she says, 'I'm Janet Smith, what's your name?'

'Lorraine,' I mutter. The girl looks me up and down and I begin to feel uncomfortable.

'I'm the second oldest in the family,' says Janet Smith. She tosses back her hair with an air of importance. 'How old are you?' she says.

'Oh, I'm eleven,' I mutter.

'Well I'm twelve, says Janet Smith, 'thirteen in two months.'

I half smile at her.

'This here's my big brother,' says Janet. 'He's nearly fourteen.'

A tall skinny boy looks my way and scowls at me.

'He's the oldest,' says Janet, 'and his name is Trevor.'

She then points to two kids fighting on the floor, 'That's our Jimmy and Julie,' she says. 'Don't mind them; they are always skylarking about.'

A little girl walks up to us and Janet picks her up in her arms. 'This is our little sister Emma,' she says, 'and she's nearly four.' Janet wrinkles her nose. 'Pooh, you stink,' she says, putting Emma back down. 'Mam, Emma needs her nappy changing again.' Mrs smith smiles. 'I'll see to her in a second,' she says.

'But Mam, she stinks, she did it ages ago.'

'Well why didn't you see to her?' says Mrs Smith.

'There aren't any clean nappies' says Janet.

I look on, shocked.

'What's wrong?' says Janet,

'My little brother was using his potty by the time he was two,' I say.

'So what?' says Janet. 'Our Emma won't go on the potty.'

'But you said she's nearly four. Our Michael uses the toilet now and he's only three.'

'Well what one kid will do another one won't,' says Mrs Smith, scooping Emma in her arms.

Four boys sit at the table playing snap.

'You're cheating !' shouts one of them.

'No I'm not.'

'You are.'

'Stop arguing,' says Janet. She then turns to me.

'That's Shane, Bob, Frank and Jimmy. They've been staying with us for two weeks now but today they're going back home to Leeds.'

At this moment a boy of about six and a little girl walk through the door. 'And this is our Paul and Tony, they're my brothers.'

'How many brothers and sisters have you got?' I ask.

'Three brothers and three sisters,' says Janet, 'and I'm the second oldest.'

'I know, you told me' I reply.

'I think it's time you all went out to play,' says Mrs Smith.

'Take Grahame and Lorraine to the park,' she says.

'But I want to go on the beach,' says Grahame in a small voice.

'We're not allowed to go on our own,' says Janet. 'Not while you're staying.'

Mrs Smith sighs. 'I'm busy right now,' she says, 'I'll take you another day.'

We leave the house and walk to the end of the street. Janet takes us into a field which has a slide, a set of swings and a witch's hat roundabout. I sit on one of the swings and Grahame sits on the one next to it. After about an hour I start to get a bit fed up of the park.

'Can we go to the amusements now?' I ask.

Janet looks at me as though I'm a bit silly.

'And where do you think we're going to get the money from?'

'Ask your Mam' says Grahame.

Janet laughs. 'Me Mam ain't got any money,' she says. 'Why do you think she lets all you kids stay at our house?'

'What do you mean?' I ask in a small puzzled voice.

'Well,' says Janet 'she gets money from the welfare for looking after you.'

'Well can we ask her for some of that then so that we can go to the amusements?'

Janet laughs,. 'I don't think so, and anyway we have to stay in the park all day.'

.'But it's boring,' says Grahame. 'I want to go home.'

'Well you can't, you're here for the week and that's that,' says Janet. 'And you will have to get used to this park because you will be spending a long time in it.'

And we did; we must have stayed about four hours in the park before we went back to the house for our tea. It was the longest four hours of my life. The swings were too babyish and I wasn't quite tall enough to reach the witch's hat.

It's teatime and stew and dumplings is on the menu. Despite being very hungry I can't eat it, for every time I try to swallow it I gag. It isn't very nice, just a pale brown gravy consisting of a few bits of potato and diced carrot. At the bottom of the bowl is a grey thing. I think it's a dumpling and a sliver of fatty meat floats on the top.
'Don't you want your tea?' says Mr Smith.
I shake my head and despite the growling in my stomach I push the bowl away.
'More for them that does then,' says Mrs Smith as she takes my bowl of stew away and scrapes it back into the large pan standing on top of the oven.

The next four days are the same. As soon as we have eaten breakfast we are sent out to play in the park. However, this morning we are finally going to the beach.
Mrs Smith has packed some sandwiches and a large bottle of water. We arrive at the beach. The sun is hot and the water glistens temptingly.
Grahame rolls up his trousers and I begin to tuck my dress in my knickers.
'What are you doing?' says Mrs Smith.
'We're going for a paddle,' I say.
'You're certainly not; you're not allowed to go in the water.'
Grahame sighs disappointedly.
'I don't care,' says Mrs Smith. 'You can stay here and build sandcastles or something.'
'Sandcastles, but….'
'Yes,' says Mrs Smith 'because I for one am not going into the sea to pull you out if you get into difficulties, so think yourself lucky I've brought you to the beach at all.. Anyway,' she went on, 'I've got a big surprise for you on your last night.'
Grahame and I look at each other wondering what the surprise might be.
We stay on the beach for about an hour and then Mrs Smith takes us all back to the house. Grahame has a sad look on his face. "I want to go home,' he mutters to me as we walk on behind the others, 'I hate it here.'
'It won't be long now,' I say, 'only three more days. We'll be home on Sunday.'

'I know,' said Grahame, 'but school starts on Monday.' Grahame kicks a tin can that's been lying near the road. 'Fancy having to spend the last week of the school holidays here' he says.
'Never mind Grahame,' I say, trying to cheer him up But the thought of going back to school scares me a bit because when we go back it will be my turn to start senior school. South Holderness seems enormous compared with the small junior school I was used to; and the thought of starting such a big school fills me with dread.

Chapter 25

'Do you want to go and see your mum and dad today?' asks Mrs
Smith, 'I bet your Mam's missing you.'
I nod my head excitedly.
'Well we'll just go and see them for a few hours. You've only got
three days left with us before you go home anyway. But don't
forget, we have a nice surprise for you on your last night.'
Three days to me seems like a lifetime. I couldn't wait to go home
for good, play with my little brothers and sleep in my own bed. But
I can't help but wonder just what the surprise is.

We jump into Mr Smith's car and we set off for Hedon.
Eventually we get to the bottom of the lane.
'Is this where you live?' says Janet as the car bumps over the
potholes.
'My car springs…' says Mr Smith.
'This is our lane,' I say proudly.
'Well it's more like a dirt track,' says Mrs Smith as the dust flies into
the car windscreen.
'And those funny little houses; do you actually live in one of them?'
smirks Trevor.
'Get lost you,' I say to Trevor.
'They're more like shacks,' says Trevor.
Mr and Mrs Smith talk quietly between themselves and very soon
we reach Mayfield Villa.
'We're here!' shouts Grahame.
Mr Smith grinds the car to a halt. We all get out and make our way
down the long path.
Grahame runs on in front, happy to be going home for a little while.
My Mam comes home to meet us. She is wearing a blue pinny with
red flowers on it, the one I bought her for Christmas.,
She puts her arm around me and gives me a big kiss. 'Hello love,'
she says.
'They've been ever so good,' says Mrs Smith.
My Mam's face is beaming as together we all walk into the house.

'Go and have a look at your bedroom,' says my Mam.
I walk in the bedroom and I'm greeted with a set of bunk beds
which have been built into the wall.

'Look what your dad's made you,' says my Mam.
'Oh great,' says Grahame ,'I've always wanted bunk beds.'
Later on my Mam makes Mr and Mrs Smith a cup of tea.
'Why don't you all go out and play?' says Mrs Smith, settling down
to drink her tea.

'Come on Lorraine, let's go for a walk on the drain bank,' says
Grahame.
The other kids stay in the garden and Grahame and I clamber on to
the drain bank.
We walk along for some time. The sun is out and the brambles are
ripe and ready for picking, I pick one and let the juice run down my
chin.
My mouth waters at the thought of my Mam's bramble pie and
custard.
'I wish we didn't have to go back with the Smiths,' I say.
Grahame looks thoughtful. 'We could just carry on walking,' he
says 'and not go back at all.'
'No, my Mam would worry if we did that, and besides, we would
get into a lot of trouble.' I pick another bramble and pop it into my
mouth, savouring the sweet taste of late summer.
'You're right,' says Grahame, 'I suppose we had better head back.'
Reluctantly we turn around and make our way back home.
They're waiting for us when we arrive back.
'Come on,' says Mr Smith looking at his watch, 'say goodbye to your
Mam, it's time we were on our way back to Withernsea.'

I bite my lip to stop the tears from falling and look out of the car
window. My Mam stands at the gate waving. I wave back until I can
no longer see her.

We arrive back at the Smiths and reluctantly I climb out of the car.
'You kids can all go and play in the park while I get tea ready,' says
Mrs Smith.

The park is full of kids. Three boys run up to Trevor.
'Where have you been all day Trev?' says one of them.
'I've been to Hedon, to their house,' says Trevor, looking at me and
Grahame.
Trevor smirks. 'Well it's not really a house, it's more like a shack.'
'The two kids snigger. 'A shack?'

'Yeah,' says Trevor, 'they live in a little wooden shack down a filthy old dirt track.'

'No we don't, we live down the lane in a nice yellow bungalow,' I say, bursting into tears.'

'You live in a wooden hut.' Trevor laughs and the other kids join in with him.

'Well,' I say in between sobs, 'our home may be small and made of wood but at least it doesn't stink of shit like yours does.'

At this Trevor balls his hand into a fist and punches me hard in the stomach, taking my breath away. I fall to the ground. He is just about to kick me when Grahame runs over. 'Leave my little sister alone!' shouts Grahame.

'Why, what are you going to do about it if I don't?' sneers Trevor.

I struggle to my feet. Trevor is about a head taller than Grahame. Trevor glares at Grahame.

'If you don't leave her alone there'll be trouble,' says Grahame, his face turning red with fury.

Trevor laughs and at the moment Grahame rains punches on Trevor's face and neck. I have never seen Grahame so mad as he kicks Trevor. Trevor covers up his face and Grahame carries on kicking and punching him until Trevor falls to the ground.

Trevor sits hunched on the grass. His face is bleeding and he is clutching his side.

'You touch my little sister ever again and I'll bloody well kill you!' shouts Grahame.

Trevor doesn't say anything.

Grahame puts his arm on my shoulders and we walk away. The other kids look on in awe. I don't think they like that Trevor much either.

I walk on air back to the swings feeling so proud of my big brother.

That night lying in bed I go over the events of the day. It was so nice seeing my Mam and I can't wait to go home for good. Just two more days left with the Smiths, I console myself. I can hear Grahame snoring in the bed near the wall but sleep won't come for me. I don't feel very well and my stomach still aches from where Trevor punched me. I lie there in the dark room and feel salty tears running down my cheeks.

Chapter 26

'Just think,' says Grahame, 'we've been here nearly a whole week and we have only been to the beach once.' Grahame sighs.
'I know, and then we weren't even allowed to go for a paddle,' I mutter
'Never mind.' A smile appears on my brother's face. 'It's our last day today.'
'I know, I can't wait to go home tomorrow,'
'I'm sick of the bloody Smiths and I'm sick of this bloody park,' says Grahame.
'Every day's been the same,' I say. 'But just think, tomorrow at this time we will be back at home down the lane.'
We sit on the grass by the swings watching the other kids on the roundabout.
'I wonder what the surprise is. Mrs Smith says we're going to get it tonight,' I say as I thread a daisy chain.
Grahame looks on puzzled. 'Well we've waited long enough for it' he says. 'I'd love to know what it is though.'
The day passes uneventfully and soon it's time for tea..
'It's bath and an early night tonight,' says Mrs Smith.
'What about the surprise?' says Grahame.
'Oh, you'll have to wait and see,' says Mrs Smith with a smile on her face.
Not long after our bath we're sent to bed.
'Fancy having to go to bed this early,' mutters Grahame in the dark, 'we didn't even get the surprise.'
'She must have been lying to us. I bet there wasn't even going to be a surprise.'
'I can't sleep,' says Grahame.
'No, neither can I, but we'd best try because the quicker we get to sleep, the quicker morning will be here and we will be going home at long last.'
'Let's not talk any more then,' says Grahame, 'and try really hard to sleep.'
We lie there in silence for quite some time. I know Grahame isn't sleeping because he isn't snoring. Presently we hear footsteps on the stairs and Mrs Smith opens our bedroom door and flicks on the light.
'Would you like to see your surprise now?' she asks smiling. 'Come

on, get out of bed and follow me.'

Dressed in our pyjamas we follow Mrs Smith up the second flight of stairs until we reach the top of the house.. Mrs Smith then opens a bedroom door and beckons us to the window. We stand by the window and Mrs Smith opens the curtains.

'Just look at that then,' she says in a whisper.

At first I'm not sure what it is I'm supposed to be looking at. I turn to Grahame and he has also looks puzzled.

'There now, doesn't it look lovely?' says Mrs Smith.

We follow Mrs Smith's gaze as she looks at the lighthouse.

After a few minutes Mrs Smith quickly closes the curtains.

'Let's have you both back to bed,' says Mrs Smith. 'You've both had plenty of excitement.'

'Bloody hell, was that it?' says Grahame as we lie in bed. 'Some bloody surprise that was, the flaming lighthouse.' Grahame sighs disappointedly.

'Never mind Grahame,' I say, 'we're going home in the morning.'

'Thank Christ for that,' mutters Grahame.

The next morning dawns bright and early. I'm woken up by Grahame jumping up and down on his bed. 'We're going home, we're going home,' he sings excitedly.

We both get dressed quickly and go down the stairs.

'Oh, you're early birds, this morning,' says Mrs Smith as she changes Emma's nappy. Emma has messed herself again and the smell is making me feel sick.

'God, it's all up your back,' says Mrs Smith to Emma.

At that moment the toast pops out of the toaster. Mrs Smith finishes cleaning Emma's backside then stands her on the floor. She then snatches the toast from the toaster.

'Do you want a slice of toast?' she asks.

'No thank you Mrs Smith,' I reply 'I'm not very hungry.'

Eventually the other kids get up.

'Now I'm leaving you in charge, Trevor,' says Mrs Smith, 'because your father and I are just popping to Hedon to take Grahame and Lorraine home.' Mrs Smith stares at Trevor's swollen cheek bone. 'Now be good,' she says, 'and no fighting.'

Grahame and I happily say our goodbyes and make our way to the car.

We sit at the back and Mr Smith revs up the engine.

'Damn car won't start,' he mutters.

My heart sinks. 'We erm could get a taxi home,' I muster.

Mrs Smith glares at me as though I'm stupid.

'Taxis cost money,' she snaps. 'Lots of money.'

After what seems like an eternity the engine sparks into life. I give a big sigh of relief as the car chugs on.

Grahame and I look at each other and grin excitedly.

Chapter 27

My Mam is waiting for us by the gate. The Smiths drop us off, say their goodbyes and leave.
'Oh, I have missed you both,' says my Mam, giving me a cuddle.
We walk up the path happily. Our little Michael is playing in the garden and when he sees me and Grahame his big blue eyes light up. He comes running up to meet us.
I pick him up into my arms and place a kiss on his little freckled face.
'Naney Naney,' he says. 'You come back! You come back!'
'He's missed you too,' says my Mam.
We walk into the house. Baby David is sitting playing with his toys. He looks up when we walk in and smiles at us. David will be one year in a few days time. He is already walking and trying to talk. I can't believe how fast his first year has gone by.

'Did you have a nice time then?' asks my Mam.
Me and Grahame look at each other, not knowing what to say.
Grahame suddenly smiles and nods his head, 'Yeah Mam, it was great,' he says.
'Yeah,we had a lovely time,' I say quickly, hoping my Mam can't see through our lie.
'Well that's good,' says my Mam.
'I'm going for a walk,' says Grahame.
'Already? You've just come home.'
Grahame sighs. 'Well it's school in morning and I want to make the most of our last day.'
'Off you go then.'
With that Grahame disappears outside the door.

My Mam turns to me. 'Just think,' she says, 'you'll be off to Senior School in the morning.'
'I know,' I mutter.
'What's wrong? Don't you want to go?'
'I dunno.'
'Oh, don't worry,' says my Mam. 'It's going to be a bit strange, a new school and everything, but I bet you'll love it. I've got your uniform ready.' My Mam's face clouds over a little. 'Now I haven't been able to afford to get you everything new, what with your dad

not working and things, but I've made you this." She then shows me a skirt which has the hem all hanging down. 'I made it meself,' she says proudly. 'I just need to turn and sew the hem but I thought it best you try it on first and then I'll get a good idea how long you need it.'

I pick the navy blue skirt up and slip it on.

'Stand still while I pin it up' says my Mam. She then folds the skirt to the desired length and then begins to pin it up.

'Ouch!' I shout as a pin scratches my skin.

'Keep still,' says my Mam. 'I've got to get this hem straight or else it won't hang right. The skirt's all pinned up; my Mam inspects her work.

'Well, it's a bit long,' she says almost to herself, ' but it will fit you for a while.'

I look down at the navy blue skirt. It is just a simple straight one. I wanted one with pleats which stick out, but I don't like to say anything so I just smile.

My Mam then goes into her bedroom and reappears carrying the rest of my uniform.

She shows me two blouses, one white and the other pale blue. 'I managed to get you these,' she says. ' They might be a bit big but they will last you.'

I put one of them on with my pinned up skirt. My Mam folds the cuffs over and over and then fastens a blue and white striped tie around my neck.

'Oh you look so grown up, now try this on.' As I put on the grey jumper I can't help but notice it has a name tag neatly sewn on the inside with someone else's name on it. But fortunately it fits just right.

'Now try this on,' says my Mam, passing me a navy blue gabardine mac.

I look at it in horror. It has a stupid hood and looks like something that one of the Four Mary's out of my Bunty Comic would wear.

'But Mam, I can't wear that thing, it's old fashioned,' I protest.

'It's a good top coat and it'll keep you warm when your walking all that way to school.' My Mam shows me the inside. 'Look,' she says, 'it's lined. It was a bargain an' all, only cost me two bob and it's hardly ever been worn.'

'I'm not at all surprised,' I say.

'Anyway, you'll have to wear it, your old coat's hardly fit for the rag bag,' says my Mam, ignoring my comment.

'Come on, try it on.'

Reluctantly I put on the offending coat. Yet again it's far too big. The pockets which should reach my waist end somewhere near my knees.

'But Mam, it's far too big.'

'It just wants the hem turning up,' says my Mam. 'We can let it down as you grow. You should get a few winters out of it.'

'But I hate it. It's not fair, why can't I have a new uniform like our Grahame did?'

My Mam rolls her eyes to the ceiling and looks a bit upset.

'I've told you Lorraine,' she says slowly, 'I just can't afford it this year.'

I look at my Mam. She looks sad like she's going to burst into tears.

'Look, I've tried my best love.' Her bottom lip wobbles. 'But it's just not easy, you know.'

I start to feel a bit mean for upsetting my Mam because I know she's tried her best and it's not her fault my dad isn't working.

I force a smile on my face. 'I didn't mean it Mam,' I say, 'it's erm a lovely coat.'

My Mam brightens up a little and shows me a small brown case. 'I've got you this for your books.' she says.

'For my books?'

'Yes for your books, don't you like it?'

'Oh yeah, it's fine Mam,' I lie, trying to keep the disappointment from showing in my face; because I really want a satchel, a real leather satchel with shiny buckles on the strap like all the other kids have.

I have been lying awake in my bed for ages. I'm filled with a mixture of excitement and apprehension at the thought of starting South Holderness school in the morning.

It will seem very strange to be starting all over again because I will be one of the youngest kids in the school, no longer in the top class like I was in Juniors.

My mind is full of what ifs? *What if I get bullied? What if they call me names? What if the teachers are all horrible? What if the work's too hard,* and on and on it goes round and round in my head. I know I need to sleep but the more I try the harder it is. So I put my head beneath my covers and flick on my torch. I reach for my comic from under my pillow and try to read in the flickering light. The Four Mary's are on the first page, reminding me of that horrible coat, so I cross my fingers hoping that tomorrow will be sunny then at least I won't be expected to wear the thing on my first day.

Sighing I throw the Bunty comic out of bed and decide to change it for the JACKIE magazine.

****

'Lorraine, come on, it's time you were up.' says my Mam.

I open my eyes. It seems like I have only been sleeping for a little while.

'Come on now, you don't want to be late on your first day do you?'

I slowly get out of bed.

'That's a good lass, now have a little wash and after you've had your toast and tea you can put on your school uniform.'

My heart sinks.

I go to the sink and pour the hot water from the kettle into a bowl, mix it with the cold and wash my hands and face. Then I force down a mouthful of toast.

'Aren't you going to eat the rest?' says my Mam.

'I'm not very hungry,' I reply in a small voice.

'It's just your nerves love,' says my Mam. 'It's a big day for you, starting a new school, but don't worry, you'll be all right when you get there, I bet you'll love it.'

I sigh, wishing I could share her enthusiasm.

I open my case. My P.E kit is neatly folded up at the bottom.

'I've put that in for you,' says my Mam, 'just in case you're doing it today.

Have you got your crayons and pencils?'

'Yes Mam.'

'And your new pen?'

I nod my head and smile. I like my new pen. It is a fountain pen with a silver nib which you fill with ink, it is much posher than an ordinary biro and I can't wait to use it.

I had seen Grahame writing with his and the writing seemed so neat and just seemed to flow off the page.

'Off you go then,' smiles my Mam looking at the clock. 'You want to be there in plenty of time on your first day.'

'Bye then Mam,' I say

'Don't forget your coat, it might rain.' My Mam hands me the gabardine mac.

Hesitantly I put it on.

'See you love, and don't worry.' says my Mam.

As soon as I am outside I take the mac off and carry it over my arm. Then I set off on the two mile walk to South Holderness School in Preston.

Chapter 28

We are led into the big school hall. The first years are told to sit on the front rows facing the stage. I sit down next to Pat. She looks as nervous as I feel.

The teachers sit on the stage, apart from one dressed in a black flowing robe who is standing in the centre. He speaks into a microphone.

'Can you all be seated as quickly as possible?' he says.

Only a clatter of chairs can be heard in the school hall as the kids sit down.

The teacher waits until everyone has sat down, then he begins his speech.

'We would like to welcome you all back to school,' he says without smiling.

He then casts his eyes at the front rows. 'And most of all,' he says, 'we would like you to welcome the first years and help them all you can, because don't forget you were all first year once.'

After the assembly the teacher addresses the front rows. 'Now will all the first years remain seated,' he says, 'and then I will call out everyone's name and tell them whose form they are in.' The teacher looks at the papers in front of him and begins to call out names. Eventually he calls my name and tells me that I'm in Strickland and that my house colour is green and my form teacher is called Mr Long. I wait for him to call out Pat's name but he doesn't and I begin to feel a bit sad because we will no longer be in the same form. After the teacher has called out everyone's name and told them which form we will be in we are told to leave the hall.

'Will all of Strickland please form a line,' says a teacher with black hair. He then introduces himself to us. 'Now I'm Mr Long,' he says, 'your form teacher. Can you please follow me to room 12B '. We follow Mr Long up a flight of stairs and walk down the corridor until we reach room 12B.

Mr Long opens the door and we follow him into the form room.

'Sit down,' says Mr Long. as he shuffles some papers on his desk.

I sit at a desk near the back and a dark haired girl sits near me.

'You're not here to bloody stop you know' hisses a boy sitting opposite me.

Others in the class notice the small suitcase by my side and start to laugh.

The girl sitting next to me smiles sympathetically. 'Take no notice of them,' she mutters.

Mr Long opens the register. 'I'll have silence,' he says. He then begins to call out our names. I discover that the girl sitting next to me is called Anne.

After Mr Long has called the register he hands out slips of paper to each of us.

'This is your timetable,' he says, 'I want you all to fill it in.' He points to the blackboard where the timetable is drawn. 'Each square represents a lesson and the room number where the lesson is held,' he says.

'And as you can see Maths is your first lesson, in room 5a, then history in room 26 and so on. Can you please copy it down?'

It all seems a bit daunting; all these lessons, all the different subjects, and how were we to know where the rooms were?

'It may take you a little while to find your way around the school,' says Mr Long as though reading my thoughts, 'but don't be afraid to ask other the older pupils, I'm sure they will help you.' Mr long then gives us a sheet of paper covered in writing.

'Now these are the school rules,' he says, 'you must read them and abide by them at all times.'

The school bell rings in my ears signalling the end of registration. There is a clatter of chairs as everyone stands up. We leave the form room and make our way to room 5a.

Anne and I stand in the corridor. She is about the same size as me. The other kids in our form are a head taller. Anne turns to me and smiles. 'I think room 5a must be downstairs,' she says. We return down the stairs and look down every corridor but we can't find the room.

'We're going to be late for the lesson,' says Anne, looking worried.

A teacher passes by. 'Are you lost girls?' he says in a booming voice.

'Yes, we can't find room 5a,' I say.

'You can't find room 5a Sir,' says the teacher sternly.

'Sorry,' I mutter, 'I mean we can't find room 5a Sir,' I stammer.

'Well you need to be on the second floor. It's the on the first corridor to the left.'

Anne and I run down the corridor towards the stairs.

'Come back here right now!' shouts the teacher.

We stop in our tracks and walk back towards the teacher who is standing there with a very angry look on his face. 'Have you read the school rules?' he bellows.

I shake my head.

'Well you if you read them you will discover that there is no running allowed in the corridors.'

'Sorry,' mutters Anne

'Sorry Sir,' says the teacher.

Anne and I look at each other. 'Sorry Sir,' we both mutter in unison.

'Now go on your way, but the next time I catch either of you running down the corridors you will get put on report.' Looking pleased with himself the teacher storms off.

We finally find room 5a. We are the last to arrive. The maths teacher glares at us as we enter the classroom. 'You're very late for the lesson,' he says.

'We got lost Sir.'

The other kids in the class titter.

'Well you had both better sit down,' says the teacher impatiently, 'we don't want to be wasting any more time.'

We sit down at a desk near the window.

'Now I want you all to turn to page seven,' says the teacher.

'Sir, we haven't got a book,' I say in a small voice.

Sighing loudly the teacher hands us a text book and a green exercise book. 'My name is Mr Waters,' he says. 'Please don't call me sir, I haven't been knighted or anything like that.'

I look on, feeling confused.

'Now write your name and form on your exercise book and then please will you turn to page seven in your text book . Mr Waters walks away. Sighing, he sits back at his desk.

I take my fountain pen and begin to write my name on the front of the book. There is a burst of ink from the pen and to my horror my new book is covered in huge ink blots. Taking a tissue I try to wipe it off but all I'm left with are big ugly smears all over the front of my book. I write down my name and form but I can hardly make out my name because of the spilt ink.

I then turn to page seven in my text book. 'Algebra'; the word jumps out at me. We did a little bit of Algebra in the junior school and I hated it. I was never very good at it.

'Now I want you to answer the set questions,' says Mr Waters.

I didn't understand the questions, never mind knowing what the answers are. They might as well have been written in Arabic as far as I was concerned.

I guess at some of the answers then I spend most of the one hour lesson trying to mop up the ink blots that had spewed on to my page.

'I think your pressing too hard on your pen,' mutters Anne.

I look over at Anne's work and notice that she hadn't written many answers down either.

A boy is asked to collect up the books. To my relief the lesson is over. The bell goes and we make our way to the next lesson which is P.E.

'Your not wearing the correct P.E kit,' says the teacher, singling me out in front of the whole class.

'You need a proper blouse not just a T shirt, and those shorts are not proper school shorts; they need to be in navy blue not black.' The teacher looks at me disdainfully.

'Have you brought your hockey boots?' she asks as though she already knows the answer.

I shake my head, 'I haven't got any Miss,' I say.

'Well make sure you do for next week. Your parents have had plenty of time to get you the correct P.E gear.' With her head in the air the teacher walks away, and I know that I'm not going to like her very much.

The rest of the day goes by in much the same way. I keep on getting lost and am told to stay behind at break time for been late for history. I make up my mind there and then that I don't like this school very much at all.

I walk home with Claire and Pat. Claire is a second year now.

'I haven't had a very first good day. I hope it gets better,' I say.

Claire tosses her hair back and laughs. 'It gets worse,' she says.

I groan inwardly and begin to wish I was back at primary school.

'How was your day Pat?' I ask.

'It was all right,' says Pat with a smile. 'I made lot's of new friends.'

My stomach sinks to my feet. Pat turns to me. 'Have you made any new friends?' she asks.

'No not really,' I reply sulkily, 'apart from one a girl I sit near; she seems all right.'

'Tell you what,' says Claire smiling, 'do you want to meet me at break tomorrow?'

'That will be great,' I say, 'where shall I meet you?'

'Meet me at morning break in smokers' corner.'

'Smokers' corner?'

Claire laughs. 'You mean you have been at the school for a full day and you don't know where smokers' corner is?'
I shrug my shoulders, feeling puzzled. Claire takes a cig from her satchel, strikes a match and lights it up.
'Smokers' corner is just by the domestic science and the sewing rooms,' she says through a cloud of smoke. 'It's a little corner in the main playground away from the bloody teachers.'
Claire cups the cig in her hand. 'Do you wanna drag?' she says.
Some big kids walk by and I can't help but notice that they are also smoking.
I take the offered cig off Claire and casually put it to my lips. The smoke burns my throat and I start to feel a bit sick.
Claire takes the cig back off me and carries on smoking it.
'Did you like that?' she asks.
'Yeah, it was all right,' I say in between coughs.
'Have you got any homework?' asks Pat.
'Not much. I've just got to back my exercise books.'
It's now Pat's turn for a drag of the cig. She laughs as she takes it from Claire.
She takes a short drag and gives the cig back to Claire.
We walk on until Pat goes her separate way to her home.
'See you in morning,' I say.
'Are you meeting me and Lorraine at break tomorrow?' says Claire.
'Dunno,' says Pat as she walks off towards her home.

'Do you like your new school?' says my Mam as I walk through the door.
'Yeah, it's all right Mam' I lie.

******

'Whose the little 'un, she only looks about nine' says a lanky boy taking a drag of his cig.
'It's Lorraine, she's me mate, gis a drag of your cig.'
The boy hands Claire his cig and she takes a long drag. 'Can me mate have a drag?' she says.
'Yeah, you might as well share it, I've got plenty.' The boy takes a packet of cigs from his pocket, takes one out and lights it up.
I take a drag of the cig and I feel really important standing here with all the big kids smoking like an adult.

'You a first year?' says a girl wearing red lipstick and a skirt hitched well above her knees.

I nod my head.

'We don't usually let first years in smokers' corner,' she pouts.

'Lorraine's all right, she won't say nowt,' says Claire.

The girl looks me up and down. 'How long have you been smoking?' she asks.

'Oh ages,' butts in Claire.

'Is that what's stunted your growth?' she laughs.

I shrug my shoulders. 'It might be,' I say, joining in her laughter.

Suddenly the boy who has been on look out pokes his head around the corner.

'Teachers!' he shouts.

We drop our cigs and make a hasty dash from the corner and scatter into the playground.

'That was a narrow escape,' says Claire.

I nod my head in agreement.

The whistle blows. 'See you at dinner time in the corner,' laughs Claire as we all go back into the school and on to our next lesson.

Over the next two weeks I come to the conclusion that I'm never going to like South Holderness school. To my horror I discover that I have to go to the remedial class for Maths. I feel ashamed because it is known as the dunces' class. However, the work is a lot easier; no more algebra or fractions, just very basic arithmetic, some of which I had already done in the infants school.

I'm always in trouble for not having the correct school uniform or P.E kit. And I'm often told off for not combing my hair as it is always sticking up. This is not my fault; I do comb my hair but it's fine and flyaway and always looks a mess. I'll never forget the day the headmistress marched me to her office and brushed my hair.

Apart from Anne I haven't made many new friends and I often get teased by the other kids which leads to me retaliating and getting into fights. I'm always in trouble for this. However, I love standing in smokers' corner with the big kids, listening to their jokes and joining in with their swearing and smoking. I feel accepted there and so grown up.

I no longer buy sweets with my pocket money and any other money I get I spend on cigarettes. I sometimes steal them from my Mam but I don't like doing this very much and only do it when I'm desperate. I hide them beneath the bushes down our path. Pat has also started smoking and on a night after school we buy five Park Drives between us. We have two cigs each and save one which we share on the way to school the next morning.

Chapter 29

The chemistry lab stinks of rotten eggs and sulphur. Our teacher Mr Winters has a black beard and wears glasses on the tip of his nose. There are no desks in the chemistry lab, just big tables and stools. I sit at the back out of sight. The teacher points to the blackboard

'This lesson I want you all to read what's written down and copy it into your book,' he says.

I look at the blackboard and can hardly make out a word of what it says in the small scrawly writing. So I just sit and do nothing and wait for the lesson to finish.

After half an hour and much to my relief the bell goes, signalling the end of the last lesson of the day.

'You have not done one scrap of work in the whole lesson!' shouts Mr Winters peering over my shoulder and looking at my exercise book.

I shrug my shoulders. "So what?' I say.

Mr Winter's face turns purple. 'You lazy, insolent girl!' he shouts. He then gives me a piece of paper. 'It's lines for you,' he says. 'You can stay behind and write five hundred times 'I must respect my teachers at all times'. And don't think you are leaving this class until you have written every one.' Mr Winters sits down at his desk and orders me to sit at the front.

The other kids smirk at me as they walk by.

I stare at the blank papers in front of me. Picking up my pen I slowly begin to write.

Mr Winters glares at me from his desk and his eyes speak of his fury.

After what seems like ages I finish the boring task and stand up and hand the papers to Mr Winters who scrutinises my work and counts every line.

'You may go,' he says sternly, 'and let that be a lesson to you.'

Sulkily I leave the classroom.

'Where the hell have you been? I've been waiting for you for bloody ages,' says Claire.

'I got detention off old Winters,' I mutter. 'I had to do lines.'

'Bloody teachers,' said Claire.

I look around. Apart from Claire and myself the cloakroom is empty. It seems like a different place.

'Do you fancy getting your own back?' says Claire.

'My own back?'

'Yeah, on the teachers.'

I nod my head slowly. 'Come on,' says Claire, 'I know what we'll do.'

We walk into the girls' toilets. Claire starts to plug up all the sinks.

'Let's just turn the taps on and go,' she says.

I agree, laughing. We then turn all the taps on and run out of the toilets and out of the school building.

We don't stop running until we are well out of the school gates.

Claire looks at me and we both burst out laughing. I laugh until I think my sides are going to split.

As though in celebration I take a cigarette from my pencil case, light it up and then offer Claire a drag. She accepts it eagerly.

'God, them toilets will be flooded by now,' says Claire through a cloud of smoke.

'Bloody hell though, what if we get found out?' I say, beginning to feel a little worried.

'We'll only get the slipper,' says Claire. 'I've had it loads of time and it doesn't even hurt. Anyway, they can't prove it was us.'

'If my mam and dad found out they'd go up the wall,' I say.

'Oh stop fretting,' says Claire, stealing a second drag of the cigarette. 'I don't suppose your mam and dad are bothered about what you do.' Claire then hands me the cigarette back.

I snatch it off her. 'What do you mean?' I say sharply.

'Well, they don't care about you, do they?'

'They do,' I say, feeling annoyed and upset.

'I told you before,' says Claire knowingly, 'they can't do.'

'They do!' I shout, holding back my tears.

'No they don't, because if they did they would have done something when that man got you, you know that man you told me about who…'

'Shut up! You don't know anything and it's got nowt to do with you!' I shout.

'Don't tell me to shut up,' says Claire, giving me a push.

I fall to the ground, scraping my knees.

Claire stands laughing.

'You fat pig,' I say.

Claire looks furious and kicks me in the side because she hates anyone calling her fat.

My side aching, I try to stand up.

'I'm never going to be your mate again!' barks Claire.

With tears rolling down my face I struggle to my feet. Claire runs off laughing.

My case came open when I fell and my books are all spewed on the ground. My chemistry book is lying in a puddle so I know there will be more lines to do when old Winters sees the state of it. But that's the least of my troubles, because my best friend has fallen out with me and despite my protests I'm not sure if my Mam and dad do care about me. There are so many questions left unanswered.

Chapter 30

'Yesterday the caretaker had to wade into the toilets to turn off the taps which someone had left running after plugging all the sinks up.' says the headmistress who was standing at the centre of the stage.

All is quiet in the assembly hall. I feel my cheeks flame and am certain the head mistress is glaring at me.

'Now this,' goes on the headmistress in a voice that is edged with anger, 'is a very serious matter, and if anyone knows anything about it I want them to inform me immediately after this assembly. Now will you please turn to page twenty two of your hymn books.'

There is a rustle of paper as pages are turned over.

When the singing comes to an end I watch as Claire leaves her seat and walks across to the side of the stage where the headmistress is now sitting. I can't hear what is been said as Claire speaks to her.

The headmistress then returns to the centre of the stage. Her face is stern as she orders silence. A hush falls on the assembly hall,

'I would like Lorraine Tranmer to go and wait outside my office immediately after this assembly,' she says in a very grave voice.

Claire then returns to her seat. As her eyes meet mine I notice the triumphant smirk on her face. I know that I'm in deep trouble.

With legs like jelly I stand outside the headmistress' office. Claire is leaning nonchalantly on the wall opposite me. I don't speak to her and she doesn't speak to me.

After some time I hear the headmistress call my name. My stomach aches as I enter her office.

'Now I have discovered that you and and another pupil are responsible for flooding out the girls' toilets yesterday,' she says. 'And it has also come to my notice that you were on detention yesterday and in the school around the time it may have happened.'

The headmistress fixes me with an icy stare.

'Now what have you got to say for yourself Tranmer?' she yells.

I look down at the floor. The headmistress follows my gaze. 'And when was the last time you polished your shoes?' she asks in disgust.

'Last night,' I mutter.

'Don't lie to me girl.'

'I did, they just get dirty walking down the lane and…'

'Don't you dare answer me back. You'renot only an insolent girl, you are also a liar, and I know it was you who were responsible for flooding the toilets.'

'I never said it wasn't,' I say on the edge of tears.

'Don't you dare speak to me like that!' The headmistress then takes out a white gym shoe from beneath her desk. Holding the shoe she gets up from her seat and points to a chair in the corner. 'Go and bend over the arm of that chair,' she says sternly.

Shaking, I do as she tells me. She hits me four times with the shoe. It hurts a little but not as much as I thought it was going to.

'Now I don't want to see you in any more trouble,' she says as I stand back up.

'Because if I do you will be punished far more severely then you have just been.'

The headmistress glares at me. 'And don't think this is the end of this,' she goes on.

'Because the headmaster has decided to write a letter to your parents informing them of your behaviour.'

I walk out of the office blinking back tears. I turn slowly when I reach the end of the corridor and watch as Claire walks into the headmistress's office.

'Where do you think you have been? You're late, the lesson began fifteen minuets ago,' says Miss Bradly, our English teacher. She looks at her watch and eyes me with contempt as she waits for my reply.

'I've been to see the headmistress.'

'In trouble I suppose,' says Miss Bradly, pecking the ceiling with her nose.

I nod my head slowly.

'Well sit down and take out your reading book, and let's not waste any more time.'

I sit down on my own at the front of the class. The seat by my side is empty as Anne is now sitting with the new girl. I'm glad it's English; it's the only lesson I look forward to. I take my reading book from my case.

'Turn to page twenty seven,' says Miss Bradly.

I turn to the required page. I'm a lot further on than this as I've been reading the book at home. It's called the Family From One End Street and tells the story of the Ruggles family. They are quite poor and have lots of children, and to make ends meet the mother does other people's washing. I enjoy reading about the Ruggles as they are an ordinary family.

'Will Keith Smith begin reading aloud to the class,' says Miss Bradly.

Keith's face turns pink as he stutters and struggles over his book. He can't read very well and some of the other kids call him a dunce. I know how he feels because of my own problem with the dreaded maths.

After some time and much to Keith's relief it is someone else's turn to read aloud.

When everyone including me has had a chance to read Miss Bradly sets our homework and the bell goes, signalling the end of the lesson. Sighing, I stand up and put my book back in my case, then with the rest of my class I leave the classroom.

I see Claire in the corridor going on to her next lesson. She walks up to me smirking.

'Why did you tell on us?' I ask her.

Claire laughs. 'So that I would get off lightly for owning up,' she says. 'Besides, it was worth it to get you into trouble.'

'It didn't bother me, it didn't even hurt.'

'It will when your Mam and dad find out,' says Claire.

'Well, your Mam and dad will find out as well, so you shouldn't have told on us.'

Claire shrugs her shoulders. 'I'm not bothered,' she says, and walks away laughing.

I walk down the corridor with my head down wishing I could be like Claire. However, the thought of my what my dad will say when he reads the letter about my exploits fill me with dread and I know my Mam is going to be very upset with me.

****

The letter arrives by first post just four days later. I hear it thump on our doormat along with a few bills and circulars. Sighing, my Mam opens the brown envelope and starts to read the contents. I can feel her eyes glaring at me. It is then that I realise what the letter is about and try to make myself scarce and edge my way towards the door.

'And where do you think you're going?' says my Mam.

I stop dead in my tracks.

'What the hell do you think you've been playing at? Do you know you have gone and got yourself suspended from school, until I write a letter to the headmaster apologising for your behaviour?'

I cringe.

'I just dread to think what your father's going to say when he finds out about this.'

I burst into tears. 'Please Mam, don't tell me dad, I'm sorry, I really am.'

My Mam stares at me long and hard with a look that is a mixture of disappointment and anger. 'You have got to promise me never ever to do anything like this again' she says in a sad voice.

'I won't Mam, honest,' I say, consumed with guilt.

'Well then I wont tell him this time, but don't you let me down now, and seeing as you have already been punished at school we'll hear no more about it.'

I breathe a sigh of relief, unable to believe I had got off so lightly.

Chapter 31

The months and years passed by through a haze of cigarette smoke and more visits to the headmistress's office. I couldn't concentrate very well in class and often found myself looking out of the classroom window or scribbling away at nothing in my notebook.

I was often in trouble. And much to mother's dismay my school reports left a lot to be desired.

I looked forward to break times. I couldn't wait to join my friends in smokers' corner and listen to their jokes while enjoying a cigarette which I'd managed to buy with my dinner money.

My dad got another job and not long after that we moved away from Bond's Street. I was sad to say goodbye to the old lane, for I knew things would never be the same again. All the dwellings were getting pulled down as the land was going to be a part of some new development. The people down the lane were given money for their land and offered a council house. My dad hung on to his land for as long as he could. Eventually he sold it privately, which enabled him to secure a mortgage on a house down Church Lane. Twenty four Church Lane seemed enormous in comparison to the small

wooden bungalow we had left behind. It had a bathroom and hot running water.

I had my very own little bedroom with a sloping ceiling which I stuck my Jackie posters on. However, I missed the freedom of the old lane, the long rambling walks along the old drain bank and the wild flowers and fields.

It was about this time that I met and fell deeply in love with Danny. We met one Sunday in Withernsea. He didn't go to the same school as me and as he lived a few miles away we only saw each other at weekends. In the week we would write to each other. How I longed for weekends so that I could see him. One Saturday afternoon we went for a walk down the old lane. Our old house was still there. We made a den in the false roof. It was our secret place. We had an old straw mattress and we would lie in each other's arms listening to Danny's transistor radio.

Then as it usually happens things came to a head. I think Danny got a bit fed up and our love like so many first loves just seemed to fizzle away to nothingness.

My thoughts of becoming a school teacher also disappeared. All I wanted was to leave school. Some days I just couldn't face going at all. I would feel physically sick at the thought of sitting in the classroom and for some reason not being able to take in what was going on or what was being said. On those days I would go to the office and get my mark, then steal back out of the school building and make my way to the disused railway line where I'd walk for hours with all sorts of mixed up thoughts running around in my head. I had a lot of unanswered questions, the biggest one being why nothing seemed to have been done when I was molested all those years ago. I knew at bottom that my parents really did care about me, however I couldn't seem to forget Claire's words and wanted to know why my experience was just shoved under the carpet, festering away inside me like a wound that refused to heal.

Chapter 32

Almost as fast as my beating heart my mind is travelling back years. I remember the good times and the bad times, but most of all I remember *him.*.

I had not thought about *him* in such a long long time. I'd refused to let the memory surface, had buried it away in a safe place so that it couldn't get out to hurt me again. But something has penetrated that safe place, for it is now open and the memories have come flooding out, taking over my mind, my every thought until the good memories, the nice ones, just seep away. I close my eyes and tightly bite my tongue hard until I can taste the warm sickly rusty flavour of blood. With my thumb I rub the skin on my arm until the skin breaks, but the soreness does nothing to blot out the memories. I want to run but I know it is pointless because *he* will still be in my head.

I can almost see him, smell the sour stale reek of his body, feel his hot fetid breath on my neck and hear the beating of my own heart.

'Lorraine, it's time to get up, you don't want to be late on your first day.'
I sit bolt upright in bed, relieved to hear my mother's voice.

'Eat some breakfast, you've got a long day of you ahead.'
I watch as my Mam pours cornflakes into a bowl. I just shake my head.
'Do you feel a bit nervous love?'
My Mam smiles gently. 'It's only natural,' she says. 'You're bound to feel a bit nervous on your first day at work. It's a big step. Come on, eat your breakfast.'
'I'm not hungry,' I mutter.
My Mam looks at me closely. 'Are you sure there isn't anything else bothering you? You have been a bit odd lately.'
I shake my head and pick up the blue and yellow overall from the back of the chair.
I put it on quickly and then step into my platform shoes.
'Don't you think you should wear something a bit more comfortable? Don't forget you will be on your feet most of the day stacking shelves in that shop.'
She hands me a pair of flat shoes and with a sigh I take off my

platforms and put them on.'

'It's for your own good lass,' says my Mam. 'You don't to want end up getting bunions on your feet like I have.'

'Bye then Mam.' I walk towards the door.

'Don't forget your sandwiches and your bus fares,' says my Mam, handing me some coins and a small bag. 'You can see me right when you get paid.'

I pick up the bag and leave the house.

'Good luck,' says my Mam as I walk through the door.

I stand at the bus stop and fasten my coat up, concealing my work uniform.

The bus pulls up and I step on to the platform.

I sit at the back on a seat near the window and listen to the school kids chatter as they travel to the posh school in the City.

'Fares please,' says the conductor stopping at my seat.

'Half to Holderness road.' I watch as the conductor clips my ticket, hoping he doesn't guess my real age.

'Back at school already,' he laughs as he hands me my ticket.

I smile, glad that I have got away with not having to pay the full fare.

I sit on the back seat and the bus speeds on.

As the bus nears my work place I begin to feel a little apprehensive.

What if I don't like my new Job, what if I can't get on with the people I'm working with, what if they don't like me, what if the work's too hard?

I then think of the six pounds ten pence I'm going to earn and it begins to burn a hole in my pocket before I get it. *Six whole pounds* I muse, *just think of the things I can buy myself with that.* Visions of records, make-up and modern clothes fill my mind. *It'll be great, all that money just for me.*

I sit by the window. Before I know it the bus pulls up at Goodfellows Supermarket, the shop where I'm going to start work.

Hesitant now, I climb off the bus and walk slowly towards the shop.

'Oh, so you're the new one. You're nice and early I see, well that's a good start.' The manageress leads me into a large storeroom at the back of the shop.

'Make yourself a cup of tea,' she says, pointing to a kettle standing on a cluttered surface. 'Have you brought your cup?'

I shake my head.

'Well, we all have our own cups here, but not to worry, you can use this one.'

The manageress hands me a blue mug.

I stand in the store room. A mixture of soapy smells fill my nostrils, making me want to sneeze.

As I wait for the kettle to boil a woman walks in. She looks me up and down.

'So you're the new lass then' she says.

'Bloody hell, you don't look old enough to be working. Either that or I'm getting older.' She hangs her coat on the peg by the wall.

Very soon the rest of the staff arrive, all wearing the same blue and yellow overalls.

'How was your weekend then Freda, did you go anywhere?'

'No, I washed me hair. Looks like you did the same by the state of your neck.'

'I like that lippy you're wearing.'

'Am I on frozen food today?'

'Dunno.'

'Come on you lot, stop your gabbing, it's time you started work' says the manageress as she walks into the storeroom. 'This is Lorraine by the way, it's her first day here so go easy on her.' She then turns to a tall black haired girl. 'Now Jane, you're on biscuits. And you can show Lorraine how to price up the tins of dog food. Carol, well you're on frozen foods.' Carol groans. 'The rest of you are on the tills. Come on then, jump to it.' The manageress snaps her fingers and the staff follow her out of the storeroom.

I stand facing the shelves of dog food.

'Are you a bit nervous?' says Becky. 'Not to worry, the work's easy enough. I'll show you how to go on.' She then hands me a list. 'Go to the warehouse just up the stairs and get two boxes of each of these and then when you have brought them all down we can price 'em up and stack 'em on the shelves. Just tell Jim, the warehouse lad, what you want. He'll sort you out.' Becky smiles.

I take the list and go to the back of the shop and up the stairs which lead to the warehouse.

'Hiya love,' says Jim. 'You the new lass?'

I nod my head and hand him the list.

'This is a shipping order,' he says as he looks at the list. 'The shelves must be almost empty.'

Jim then begins to stack boxes of dog food against the wall. He then hands me a box.

'Be careful, it's heavy.'

My arms ache as I carry the box back down the stairs and inside the shop.

'Oh, good lass,' says Becky. 'Now you can price them up. Here's your stamper.'

I pen the box and take out a tin and stamp the price on to the top.

Becky sighs. 'No not like that,' she says. 'Price them up whilst they're still in the box and then begin to fill the shelves with them. It's quicker that way.'

Becky then goes to the warehouse. When she returns I have emptied the box and have started to fill up the shelf.

'Turn the tins around so that the label faces you,' says Becky. 'That's it, good lass, I'll make a good shelf stacker out of you yet.'

The day passes and after countless more trips to the warehouse the shelves are stacked neatly.

My back aches from carrying the heavy boxes and I feel extremely tired after such a long busy day.

'Well how did it go then?' says my Mam when I walk into the house.

'It was great, much better than school, but God *I'm tired.'*

'Been working hard then?'

'You can say that again; my back's killing me.'

'I bet you're glad I told you to change out of your platforms, now aren't you?'

I nod my head and sit back on the couch. My Mam enters the kitchen and I close my eyes. The next thing I know my Mam is waking me up with a plateful of food.

'Eat your tea ,' she says. 'You need to keep your energy up.'

Chapter 33

'Have you got a light please?'
The bloke smiles at me as he hands me a box of matches. He's got shoulder length dark hair and a twinkle in his big brown eyes.
'What's your name then?' he says.
'Lorrraine' I reply as I light my cigarette, casually blowing the smoke into the atmosphere.
'That's a lovely name,' he says, smiling.
A woman standing nearby looks on.
'Been waiting long then?'
'Yeah, the bus is always late,' I say, trying to act cool.
'Where're you going?'
'Home.'
'Where's that then?'
'Hedon.'
'What you doing round here then?'
'I'm just on me way home from work. I'm a shop assistant.'
'I see,' says the bloke, eyeing my overall. 'Been working there long?'
'Oh ages,' I lie. I look up into his eyes. *God, he's gorgeous.*
'How old are you?'
'Seventeen ' I say, feeling my face going red at my lie.
'I'm twenty four,' he says, looking me up and down.
Twenty four, and he's chatting me up.
'I'm not in the habit of picking up lasses at bus stops, but there's something about you and I really want to see you again.'
He fancies me.
'Would you meet me tonight at around seven o'clock?'
'Yeah, okay,' I say, quickly forgetting to play it cool.
'That'll be great. I tell you what, you could bring a mate with you if you want and I could bring my friend. We could make a foursome.'
I think of Pat and I nod my head.
'Well, how about meeting us outside the Ganstead pub near Bilton at around seven tonight?'
'Yeah, okay then.'
He smiles a nice warm smile and cups my face in his hand.
'You're really cute you know,' he says, pecking me on my cheek.
The woman standing at the bus stop looks on disapprovingly.
A blue and yellow bus pulls up.
'This is my bus,' I say.

'Okay then see you tonight, love.'
'Oh, by the way, what's your name?'
'Andy,' he laughs.
I stand on the bus platform and wave to him until the doors close in
my face.

'He's absolutely lovely, really mature, not like them daft lads down
at the youth club.'
Pat stands on her step with her arms folded. 'How old is he then?'
she asks.
'He's twenty four.'
'Twenty four,' gasps Pat, her eyes growing wide.
'Yes twenty four, and he says he's got a friend. He says we could
make up a foursome. Do you fancy meeting them tonight outside
the Ganstead?'
Pat laughs. 'You bet I do,' she says, 'it will be a change from the
bloody youth club.'
'See you later then. I'll have me tea and change into me glad rags.'
'Okay,' Pat smiles as she closes her door.

'And just where do you think you're going?' says my Mam as I sail
into the room on a cloud of perfume.
'Oh, just going to pictures with a few friends Mam.'
'You're wearing a lot of make up aren't you? Good job your dad
ain't here, he'd go spare.'
I smile to myself because it was highly unlikely my dad would see
me because he was working away in Saudi Arabia.
'Look, make sure you're on that last but one bus. I don't want you in
late.'
'Oh Mam, I'm not a kid any more.'
'It makes no difference to me. Just see you get yourself home at a
reasonable hour.'
Sighing, I walk out of the door and slam it behind me.
Pat comes running up the road to meet me.
'If we hurry we'll catch the next bus.'
Just as we turn the corner we see the bus leaving the bus stop.
'Oh shit, we've missed it,' says Pat.
'Never mind, we can hitch. We should easily get a lift.'
We stand at the side of the road. Very soon a car pulls up and the
driver pokes his head out of the window. 'Hop in lasses!' he shouts.
'Where're you going?'

'To the Ganstead pub,' we reply in unison.

We sit in the back of the car.

'You know lasses, you want to be careful hitching lifts from strangers. Anything could happen to you.' The driver swerves to avoid a scraggy dog.

Pat nudges me and we both giggle.

The driver tuts and turns his radio up.

The car stops outside the Ganstead pub. He's standing there waiting for me.

"Has he bought a mate with him?' says Pat as we clamber out of the car.

'No, it doesn't look like it.'

Pat sighs disappointedly. 'Well I hope I don't have to play bloody gooseberry all night,' she says.

'You came then,' he says when we reach his side.

'Where's your mate then?' says Pat.

'He's coming later on. We're meeting him in town.'

We stand at the bus stop and wait for the bus to take us into town.

'I thought we could go back to my place and have a party,' mutters Andy shuffling from foot to foot.

'Oh yeah, that would be great,' I say.

I glance at Pat. She doesn't say anything, just looks on dubiously.

'He'll be bringing his mate later,' I say.

At that moment the bus arrives and we clamber on to the platform.

Andy pays the conductor our fares and the bus speeds on.

"Whereabouts is your pad Andy?' I ask.

'By the docks,' mutters Andy.

The bus stops on the edge of town.

Andy stands up. 'This is our stop,' he says.

We have been walking for about fifteen minuets when we reach the docks.

'Where's your flat then?' says Pat with a suspicious look in her eyes.

'I don't live in a flat,' mutters Andy, 'I erm, live on a barge.'

He then points towards the water. There are lots of barges moored tightly together.

'You actually live on one of them,' says Pat.

Andy nods his head. 'Just follow me' he says.

We follow Andy on to the riverside where the barges are moored.

Andy jumps on to one of the barges and we join him. He then jumps onto the next one until he reaches his barge. Holding my breath and not looking down at the water below I follow him.

His barge is moored about half way down. He takes us inside.

'Just stay here,' he mutters. 'I'll go and get my friend and bring us some bottles back for the party.' Andy disappears out of the small door.

I turn to Pat. 'Hey this is cool,' I say, 'a party on a barge, it's going to be great.'

Pat sighs and I can tell by the look on her face that she doesn't share my enthusiasm. 'I don't like him,' she says. 'I just don't trust him at all and we should go.'

'Oh don't be daft, we're gonna have a fab time.'

'I think we should leave. He could be anyone, I mean let's face it you don't even know him do you? What if he comes back with a gang of men and they rape us, we wouldn't stand a chance. And we could end up anywhere.'

I sit on the small bunk. Suddenly the realization strikes me. And the more I think about it the more convinced I become of my friend's warning. I grow afraid.

'Let's go, ' I say, my voice shaking.

Without hesitation we leave the barge and jump as fast as we can over the other barges until we reach the shore.

"We will have to just make a run for it,' says Pat. 'He could be anywhere.'

Together we flee from the docks and we don't stop running until we reach the centre of town. My breath is coming out in short gasps from running.

'We have to get home,' says Pat. 'He could be looking for us.'

We make our way to the bus station and for some reason I turn around. I can see Andy walking some distance behind us. I turn to Pat, 'Oh my God, he's behind us.'

'Has he seen us?' says Pat.

'He's walking this way,' I say to Pat in a panic.

My heart beating wildly, I run into a garage. Pat follows.

A car is standing by the petrol pumps.

'Will you give us a lift to Hedon?' I ask the man as he fills the car up.

'Well it's a bit out of my way' says the man, laughing.

'Please' I beg. 'We need to get away from here.'

'Are you in trouble?' asks the man.

'Sort of,' says Pat.

The man opens the car door and we climb inside. The man turns to us.

'I can't take you straight home,' he says. 'First I need to call in at my local, but you can come with me and wait while I have a couple of pints and pick up a packet of fags, then I promise I'll take you straight to Hedon.'

The car speeds down Hessle road and pulls to a stop outside a pub.

The barman doesn't bat an eyelid when we order our drinks. The man chats to a women sitting on a barstool. Smiling to ourselves we sit down.

'This is all right, isn't it? We got served' says Pat.

'Yeah, it's great' I say, feeling all warm and fuzzy inside after sipping my whiskey and ginger.

'He'll never find us in here.'

'No, he won't. I'm glad we got away.'

Suddenly the door opens and a gang of hippies enters the pub. They sit at the table near the corner.

'Oh look, we've got new faces in the pub.' I look up. The man is wearing a pair of scruffy jeans and a patched denim jacket. He has really long hair and a small moustache.

'Fancy a drink?' he asks.

We nod our heads eagerly.

"Okay.'

We sit in the corner with the gang of hippies. As we drink whiskies the pub fills up. Very soon it's crowded.

The lights dim and someone puts a coin in the juke box. The music plays loudly.

I look towards the bar. The man who brought us here is no longer sitting there.

The drink has made me feel a little light headed and my earlier worry about getting home has vanished. All I want now is another drink.

Someone is passing a large hand rolled cig around. It smells strange, sort of musky and sweet.

Time passes and we drink more whiskey. My head feels light. Faces look towards me and laugh. I know they're laughing at me. I look quickly from left to right. The laughter echoes in my ears. I feel sick and dizzy. Standing up, I push my way through the laughing faces.

'You all right little chick?' asks a leather clad biker.

I nod my head.

The man smiles at me. I look around for Pat. She is sitting in the corner with a bloke. He has got his arm around her. They both look my way and laugh. I scurry to the toilets. Apart from a girl washing her hands the toilets are empty. But I can still hear the laughter in my head. Afraid, I lock myself in the cubicle and sit on the toilet for some time. The sweat pours down my face. I place my head in my hands to but it does nothing to drown out the high pitched laughter.

'Everyone thinks I'm stupid' I mutter to myself. After some time I stand up and walk across to the sinks where I splash cold water on my cheeks and return to the tap-room.

'Where have you been?' giggles Pat, who has disentangled herself from the bloke's arms.

I look around the tap-room. The juke box has stopped playing and a lot of people have gone.

'Stop laughing at me,' I say, with tears running down my face.

'Hey, you're paranoid,' says the biker who has followed me from the toilets. 'No one's laughing at you.'

The rest of the night passes in a haze.

A man from behind the bar looks our way. 'I want you all out of here now!' he shouts 'last orders went an hour ago.'

I stand up but my legs feel like jelly and I stumble to the floor.

The biker helps me up.

Pat and her new bloke walk me towards the door and the biker follows.

The cold air hits me as soon as we get outside. I look around for the biker's motorbike but he doesn't seem to have one. He walks by my side, slinging his arm around my shoulders. Pat and her bloke walk on in front. The biker lights a cigarette.

'My name's Rob. Are you going to tell me yours, chick?'

Without answering him I look up into the red sky. It glows brightly and I want to lose myself in it.

'Hey, what's wrong babe?' asks Rob.

I tremble. 'I dunno,' I stammer, 'I just feel...' With that my legs give way and I feel myself falling. Before my head has a chance to meet the cold grey pavement Rob picks me up and steadies me. 'You okay?'

I put my hands to my head. The laughter has faded to a dull chant.

'I can still hear them,' I mutter.

'Who?'

'Them, they're still laughing at me.'

Rob turns around. Apart from the few cars on the road the street is practically empty.

'Ain't no one about.'

'But I can hear them laughing at me.'

Rob mumbles something about me having a bad trip. I look on confused as I didn't hurt myself when I fell.

I look on in front. Pat wobbles on her high heels with her arm around her new boyfriend.

'Come on, we'll cut down here,' says Rob. 'We should be able to catch up with your friend then.'

He leads me into a narrow back alleyway which cuts between two shops. My head starts spinning and I begin to feel sick.

Rob pins me up against the wall and showers my face with his kisses. His breath reeks of stale smoke and beer. My stomach aches. His hand tugs at the waist band of my skirt and it falls to the ground. I try to push him away. He doesn't move. My stomach retches and I gag. Unable to stop myself, I throw up.

Rob wipes away the vomit on his jacket and I burst into tears.

'You okay, chick?'

'S-sorry ,' I mutter.

'It's okay. I guess you couldn't help it. Not very romantic though, is it?'

I quickly hitch up my skirt and we walk out of the alley.

'Lean on me,' says Rob. 'You should start feeling better soon.'

We leave the alley and are soon back on the main drag. Pat is walking towards me.

'Where the hell did you get to?' she says. 'You weren't there when I turned around so we thought we'd better come and find you.' She hangs on to her boyfriend's arm looking a little worried. 'I don't know how we're getting home. The last bus went ages ago.'

'I suppose you could get a cab,' drawled her boyfriend.

'Have you got any money for the fare because I'm broke?'

I then realize that I'd left my handbag containing my purse back at the pub.

I shake my head.

Pat looks at her boyfriend. 'I'm skint too,' he says.

Rob rakes around in his pocket and retrieves a handful of coppers.

'Well that won't get us very far,' says Pat.

'We could still get a cab and I could explain to the driver that we will pay when we get home and then me Mam will give me the money.'

'Won't she go mad?' Pat looks at her watch. 'Oh my God, have you any idea what time it is?'

I shrug my shoulders.

'It's two o'clock in the frigging morning. I don't know about your Mam Lorraine, but my dad's going to bloody well kill me.'

Sober now, Pat hails a black cab. It pulls up. She gives her new boyfriend a hasty peck on the cheek and we climb into the cab. Rob gets into the cab with us, 'I'll come back to your place,' he says, 'mind if I kip on your couch tonight?'

Pat quickly tells the driver where we are going. With a nod of his head he drives off.

Presently the taxi pulls up outside Pat's house and drops her off and then drives on to twenty four Church Lane.

'And where the bloody hell have you been?' says my Mam when I stagger into the house.

'Mam I need to pay the taxi driver, I erm missed the last bus home, and the taxi's waiting outside.'

'The last showing at the pictures finished at ten thirty so you'll have had plenty of time to catch that last bus.' My Mam reaches for her purse. 'And I can't understand where your money's gone, you only got paid the other day.'

I stumble back out of the door and walk towards the waiting taxi. After I've paid the driver Rob gets out of the car and together we walk into the house.

'Mam,' I say hesitantly, 'this is Rob. Is it all right if he sleeps on the couch tonight?'

My Mam tightens the belt around her dressing gown. 'You've been drinking, haven't you?' she says.

I lower my head.

'It wasn't Lorraine's fault really,' says Rob. 'Some men in the pub got her drunk. She thought she was only drinking coke but it turned out they were plying her with Rum and coke. That's when I stepped in and brought her home. I got in the taxi with her to make sure she got home safely but I'm sorry, I just didn't have enough money left to pay the fare.'

I look on feeling a little surprised that Rob had so quickly invented such lies . My Mam turns to me. 'So you've been sitting in a pub,' she says. 'Well let's hope that after tonight you have learnt your lesson. It's a good job for you your dad's away.' She then looks across at Rob. 'Thanks for bringing her home son,' she says. 'God knows what might have happened to her if you hadn't. And seeing as you've come so far out of your way you can sleep on the couch, but just for tonight mind.' My Mam shakes her head and looks at me. 'And you Madam can get yourself to bed. You've got work in morning and don't think for one minute you are having the day off.' My Mam follows me as I stumble out of the door. With her help I climb the stairs. We reach the landing. My Mam sighs.
'I want that bloke out of this house by morning,' she says.

I sit up in bed and place my hands over my aching head and rock back and forth for what seems like ages.
Mick Jagger smiles down at me from the poster on my wall. I look into his eyes and then look away quickly when his smile becomes a mocking sneer.
I flick off my night lamp and close my eyes and lie in the dark. My heart beats fast, my thoughts are racing. The events of the night are all jumbled up inside my head. I run my tongue over my parched lips, trying desperately to clear my mind of everything, but I can't seem to turn off my thoughts. I shudder as I remember the faces, the laughing faces and the screeching inside my head.

The church clock strikes five. The birds have woken up. The sounds of the dawn chorus fill my bedroom and the early morning sunlight streams through my bedroom window.
I curl up in the foetal position and feel my self surrendering to sleep. No sooner have I closed my eyes when I feel my mother shaking me.
'Come on Lorraine, it's time you were up for work.'
I groan. My head aches.
'Don't think you're having the day off,' said my Mam. 'Fancy coming in at that time when you've got work the next day. You won't do that again in a hurry, will you?'
I get out of bed and slowly dress.
'Come on, hurry up, you're going to be late.'
In the bathroom I splash cold water on my face but it doesn't cool down my flaming cheeks. My mouth feels so parched and my

stomach aches.

I walk into the living room. Rob is still asleep on the couch, his blankets in a tumbled heap.

My Mam takes me to one side. 'I want him out of the house soon as well,' she says, 'so you'd better look sharp and wake him up.'

Rob opens one eye. 'Morning,' he says.

My Mam looks at me. 'Have some breakfast, you'll feel better then' she says.

'She'd be better with a mug of black coffee,' says Grahame as he walks into the room. 'I heard you coming in late last night. I suppose you were pissed.'

Rob sits up. My brother gives him a long look and throws him his jeans which have been lying on the floor. 'I think you'd best get dressed pal and sod off,' he says.

'Don't be like that Grahame,' says me Mam. 'At least he brought our Lorraine home safe last night.'

'I bet he did,' says Grahame.

I follow my Mam into the kitchen. My head still aches and I feel terrible.

'I think I'll have the day off,' I mutter to myself.

My Mam looks up sharply.

'You're going to work,' she says. 'And let it be a lesson to you not to come home at that time and in that state again.'

I return to the living room. Rob is dressed now and putting on his jacket.

'We'll get going now,' I say.

'What, without a bite to eat?' says my Mam.

'I'll be okay Mam,' I mutter.

'Have you got your bus fares and your dinner money?'

I look in my pocket. Apart from two pence and an old receipt it is empty.

'Well you won't get very far on that.' My mam hands me some money.

'I don't know what you've done with your wages. You only got paid the other day,' she says.

'Thanks Mam, I'll pay you back at the end of the week.'

'Aye, well, see that you do lass.'

I say goodbye to my Mam, and Rob and I leave the house.

Rob puts his arm around me as we walk to the bus stop.

'How do you feel?' he asks.

'Terrible. I'm never going to drink again.'

'That's what they all say,' he laughs.

We stand at the bus stop and very soon the bus arrives.

'I have no money,' says Rob. 'Do you think you can get my fare?'

'Yeah sure,' I say, dipping into my purse, knowing that I will have to go without dinner in order to pay Rob's fare.

We sit together at the back of the bus. Rob smiles.

'You looked fantastic last night,' he says. 'I thought you were about eighteen.'

I cringe, wondering what he thinks of me now, dressed in an overall minus my make-up.

'You look all right now though,' went on Rob as though reading my thoughts.

'Will you be my bird?'

I gaze into Rob's eyes. He's quite good looking and I feel sort of protected with his arm swung over my shoulders. So I smile and nod my head.

Rob kisses me on the lips and it feels nice. I sigh, wanting it to go on forever.

An old woman sitting nearby looks on disapprovingly.

Ignoring the woman's disdainful looks Rob kisses me again. This time it's a long lingering kiss which almost takes my breath away. He holds me in his arms.

'You're such a sweet little chick,' he says.

'How old are you?' I ask, suddenly realizing that I know nothing really much about him.

'Nineteen in a couple of months,' says Rob.

His face clouds over. 'You don't think I'm too old for you do you?'

I smile and shake my head, feeling pleased with myself.

'No, of course not,' I say in a whisper.

The bus draws to halt outside the shop where I work.

'I'll see you at dinner time then,' says Rob as we step off the platform.

'Okay, see you at twelve.' I plant a kiss on his cheek and walk into the shop.

'Who was that?' says the manageress as I walk through the door.

'My new boyfriend.'

'Well I don't like the look of him. He looks like one of those Hell's Angel types.' The manageress tuts. 'Nothing but trouble if you ask me anything.'

'No one's asking you anything,' I mutter under my breath.

The manageress turns around and glares at me. 'What was that you just said?' she asks.

'Oh nothing, nothing.'

'Well it would pay you to get on with your work. You're on dog food today.'

I look at the half empty shelves which I have to fill up with tins of dog food and sigh wearily. My first job is to take stock of the tins I need to fill up the shelves. I do this slowly then go to the warehouse with my list.

'Ain't you very well?' says the warehouse lad as he piles up the boxes of tinned dog food against the wall.

I shrug my shoulders. 'I'm okay,' I mutter.

'Well you don't look it, in fact you're as white as a bottle of milk.'

'Just tired ' I say with a yawn.

'Oh, I see. Been burning the midnight oil have you?'

Ignoring him I bend down and pick up a box of tins. My legs wobble beneath me as I struggle with the box to the shop floor. I can hear the girls giggling behind the biscuit counter and I know they're laughing at me.

I slowly place the box on the floor and open it and as the place fills up with early morning shoppers. I begin to stamp the price on to the tins and slowly stack the shelves.

'Come on, hurry up,' says the supervisor. 'You'll never get finished.'

A yawn escapes from my mouth.

'My God, you've come here to work, not to day dream.' The supervisor sighs and struts on and the giggling behind the biscuit counter increases.

The morning passes with more visits to the warehouse. My back aches and I feel sick.

The humming of the cash registers fills my ears. My head aches and throbs.

I glance out of the window. I can see Rob. He is leant up against the wall with his hands in his pockets. The supervisor taps me on the back.

'He's been hanging around all morning and I don't like the look of him. He ought to get himself a job instead of picking up young lasses.' The supervisor looks at the clock.

'You can get going for your lunch hour now,' she goes on, 'but just watch what you're doing. That bloke looks far too old for you.'

I walk out of the door glad that the morning is over.

My stomach growls. I look in my purse the only money I have is my bus fare home so going to the chip shop is out of the question. Rob saunters up to meet me. He gives me a kiss on my cheek.

We sit in a bus shelter watching the rain as it splashes off the pavements. Rob puts his arm around me. People stare out at me from car windows.

I cuddle up to Rob. A woman waiting for her bus glares at Rob and clutches her shopping bag tightly to her.

The summer shower comes to an end. 'Do you fancy a walk to the park?'

I smile and nod my head and together we leave the bus shelter.

'Have you got any money I can borrow?' asks Rob. 'I've run out of smokes.'

'I've only got my bus fare home.'

'Well if you can lend it to me I will bring you it when I meet you after work tonight.'

Smiling I give Rob the last ten pence I have in my purse.

Hand in hand we walk into the park. Rob towers above me and I feel safe and protected.

We sit on the park bench. Rob takes me in his arms. 'You're the best thing that's happened to me in a long time,' he says. 'The problem is people don't understand me.'

Rob sighs, 'I was inside once you know, in borstal.'

'What did you do?' I ask, feeling a little sorry for Rob.

'Oh, I was a bad lad,' is all Rob says. 'But I had a really rough time in there.'

'What did you do?' I repeat.

'I don't like talking about it.'

I look into Rob's eyes and he looks sort of sad. 'Do you want a cig?' I ask in an effort to change the subject.

Rob takes a cig, lights it and inhales deeply. 'The problem is,' he says, 'nobody seems to understand or give a knack about me, and my old woman has just thrown me out of the house so I've nowhere to go.'

'So you've been living on the streets?'

'Well sort of,' says Rob, 'but sometimes I doss at me mate's flat.'

I look into his sad eyes and my heart goes out to him.

'I know how you feel in a way,' I mutter.

'What do you mean?'

'Well I sometimes feel that no one cares.'

'Why do you feel like that?'

'Oh, nothing.'

'There must be a reason.'

'It was just, well, something happened to me once.'

'Something bad?'

Yeah but I'm like you, I don't talk about it much.'

Rob pulls me closer to him. 'Well you're my girl now, and you can tell me everything or anything you want.'

'It was something that happened when I was about five years old, something I'll never forget.'

'And it makes you feel bad.'

'Yeah, and sort of guilty and dirty in a way.'

'Well, why don't you tell me about it? It might make you feel better.' Rob pauses. 'Yeah, you know, lighten your load a bit babe.'

'It happened a long time ago' I mutter, half to myself.

'And it still bothers you?'

'Yes. It bothers me more now then it ever has done, and if I tell you about it you might not,' I pause searching for the right words, 'like me any more' I say slowly.

'You can tell me anything, and I'll still like you. In fact I've fallen for you in a big way.'

Slowly I find myself telling him all about Ralph.

'Bloody hell,' says Rob when I finished. 'And you have kept it all to yourself all this time? No wonder you got so freaked out.'

'I told a friend once and she said that my Mam and dad don't really care about me as nothing was ever done about it, not even when I'd told my Mam.'

'Well I care about you,' says Rob, taking me in his arms, 'and I won't let anything bad happen to you ever again.'

Rob holds me tight as we walk for some time around the park. Kids are playing happily on the swings while the mothers watch them as they sit talking together on the park bench. I begin to wish I was a child again, oblivious to everything.

The mothers look my way and then begin talking to each other and I know they are talking about me.

'Do you feel okay?' asks Rob.

'I dunno,' I mutter.

'What's wrong?'

'Oh nothing, but it's time I was going back to the shop.'

'We'll get going then.'

We leave the park and on the way we share a cigarette.

'Do you like working at the shop?' asks Rob.

'It's okay, I just wish everyone would leave me alone.'

'What do you mean?'

'Well I heard them all laughing at me behind the biscuit counter.'

'Laughing at you?'

'Yes, just like all those women sitting on the bench were talking about me and saying bad things.'

Rob shook his head. 'I think you're still a bit paranoid, I never heard them say anything.'

'They did, I could tell.'

We walk along in silence. Rob puts his arm around me and I begin to feel a bit better. My stomach growls as we reach the shop.

'I'll meet you when you have finished work,' says Rob. He plants a kiss on my lips and I walk into the shop.

'You're fifteen minutes late,' said the supervisor,' looking at her watch. 'So you had better get on with your work before we dock it out of your wages.'

The afternoon passes in a haze. The laughter behind the biscuit counter increases and the ringing from the cash machines increases my splitting headache.

At last my work day is over. My legs wobble as I walk out of the shop, my stomach aches and all I want to do is get on the bus, go home and have something to quell my hunger pains and rest, perfect rest.

Rob is waiting for me outside. He walks up to me smiling and kisses me on the cheek.

'Have you got my bus fare?' I ask.

Rob looks at me quizzically.

'The ten pence you borrowed at dinner time, it was my bus fare.'

'Oh I forgot about that, sorry I ain't got a bean.'

'How am I going to get home now?' I say, a little annoyed.

'Well can't you do what you did last night, just get a cab and let your Mam pay when you get home.'

'No,' I say shaking my head, 'my Mam would go up the bloody wall.'

"Well there's nowt else for it babe, you're going to have to walk home.'

'But it's five mile away.'

'I'll come with you,' says Rob. 'Don't worry, we'll soon get there. I walk about all day long; you get used to it.

It took us two hours to walk home and by the time we reached our house my legs ached.

'Where have you been?' said my Mam. 'My God, you're as white as a bottle of milk. Sit yourself down lass, what have you been doing, working overtime?'

I nod my head quickly. 'Stock taking,' I reply.

My Mam then looks towards the door and sees Rob standing there.

'Lorraine's tired and she's having her tea now, so I think you'd be best going home,' she says.

Rob's face drops and my heart goes out to him.

'Can he stay for the night again Mam? ' I ask. 'He's homeless, his Mam's thrown him out.'

My Mam's eyes roll to the ceiling. She takes me aside. 'He can stay for just one more night, then he will have to go home and patch things up with his mother' she says.

We sit in the front room. Rob looks through my record collection and I feel my face flame when he sees my Top of the Pops collection.

'Haven't you got anything else?' he asks.

'No, sorry, I can't afford the real thing so I have to make do with those. But I have got a few forty fives. This one's my favourite, have you heard it?

'What is it?'

'It's called: Without You.'

Rob nods his head and smiles. 'Yeah, it's all right, play it if you like.'

I put the record on and we sit back on the couch.

I lay my head on Rob's shoulder as Nilsson starts to sing.

The music plays and Rob holds me tight.

We play the record several more times. My eyes begin to feel heavy.

'Can't live if living is without you, can't live can't give anymore.'

Suddenly shrieking laughter fills my head. I can no longer hear the music.

I feel someone shaking me.

I look up into Rob's eyes. 'Are you tired? You dropped off to sleep' he says.

I place my head in my arms.

'Hey, what's wrong?'

'Tell them to go away,' I say, bursting into tears.

'Tell who to go away? Ain't no one here.'

The ranting laughter becomes louder.

'There is, I can hear them, they're laughing at me.'

'You're a strange little chick, absolutely paranoid,' says Rob. 'Just relax, you're just imagining things, the mind can sometimes play strange tricks on you, especially when you're strung out.' Rob holds me to him and begins to stroke my hair until the laughter in my head fades away.

Chapter 34

My cousin and her boyfriend came yesterday. They gave me a transistor radio. It's not just an ordinary transistor, it's a special one. When I sing along with it, it broadcasts my voice and all the world can hear me singing. I've become a great singer and I know that I'm famous. Sometimes the radio plays special songs just for me. The voices I can hear inside my head tell me this. So I listen carefully to the radio all the time.

Rob is coming to see me today and together we're going to travel the world. I told my Mam all about this but she just pretended to look perplexed and said I was speaking rubbish.

She said she is taking me to see the doctor today, but he knows all about me as well because he has heard me singing on the radio.

The voices also tell me that I'm all right and that I don't have to worry about anything because it is all going to be sorted out. They tell me that I'm going to marry Rob and we are going to have a big white wedding in Hollywood and I will have one hundred bridesmaids. Pat is going to be the chief bridesmaid. I'm getting excited about my wedding because the Rolling Stones, the Beatles and Elvis Presley will be among the wedding guests and a lot of other famous people. They are all going to sing at my wedding. I just can't wait, but the voices have told me to keep it all a secret and not to spoil the surprise for my other wedding guests.

I listen to my transistor radio and lie back on my bed. My mother opens my bedroom door.

'Come on Lorraine love, I'm taking you to see the doctor.'

'Why Mam, I'm not poorly.'

My Mam looks a bit upset. 'Look Lorraine,' she says, 'you haven't exactly being yourself this last few days.'

I walk down the stairs and put on my shoes. They're my white sand shoes and I have written Rob's name all over them.

My Mam half smiles and takes my hand, which is something she hasn't done since I was little, and together we walk up the street to the doctor's surgery.

Because I'm famous the receptionist lets us go straight in to see the doctor. She gives me a knowing smile as I pass her desk.

The doctor peers at me over the top of his spectacles.

'Now Lorraine,' he says, 'why have you kept your mother up all night with your singing?'

'You want to hear me sing?'

'No, I'm sure you have a nice voice, but I just need to ask you some questions. Your mother tells me that you are behaving very strangely and that you have been talking to yourself a lot. Is this right?'

I shake my head slowly.

'You have love,' says my Mam who is sitting by my side. 'You've been talking away and singing to yourself all night.'

'I haven't, I've been talking to the others.'

'The doctor searches my face. 'What others?'

I shake my head in frustration. 'You know, the voices.'

'Voices?'

'Yes, the voices. Sometimes they laugh, sometimes they just talk.'

'But Lorraine, there was no one there,' says my Mam, 'you were talking to yourself.'

'Have you been hearing voices Lorraine? Do you know who the voices belong to?'

'The others. Do you want to come to my wedding?'

'Don't you think fifteen years old is a little young to be getting married?'

Without waiting for an answer the doctor asks me to wait in the surgery while he has a little talk to my Mam.

'There'll all waiting for me in Hollywood,' I say as I leave the room, 'I've made it right to the top.'

The doctor smiles and nods his head and I know he is as overjoyed as I am.

'You're going for a little rest,' says my Mam. 'The doctor thinks you may have been overdoing things. So we are taking you somewhere that is nice and peaceful where you will be looked after until you feel a bit better.'

'Yes,' I agree. 'A rest will do me good before I start my tour.'

My Mam sighs and shakes her head and wipes away a tear from her cheek.

I know she is sad that I'm going away.

Suddenly there is a knock on the door. My Mam goes to answer it.

I hear her talking to Rob in a low voice but I can't make out what she is saying.

I run into Rob's arms.

'Is Rob coming with me Mam?' I ask. 'Because I'm no going anywhere without him. You see we're going to get married soon.'

Rob looks on, a little surprised.

'Well I suppose he can come and see you when you're settled.'

Rob nods his head in agreement. 'I'll visit you whenever I can,' he says.

'And then when I come home we can start our tour go to Hollywood, get married...'

'Okay love, okay,' says Rob, smiling.

Chapter 35

'You won't be here for long love,' says my Mam.

I look around the room. An old lady sits rocking in her chair and a grown man sits crying.

A woman paces the floor with a worried expression etched on her grey face.

My Mam shuffles uncomfortably in her chair. She too is close to tears.

'They will be moving her to the adolescent ward as soon as there is a bed so then she will be with people more her own age' says a lady as she scribbles notes down on a piece of paper.

'While you're here love, try and get some rest and don't listen to the voices in your head because it's only your mind playing tricks on you.' My Mam kisses me on the cheek and leaves the room.

I start to cry. I don't like it here, it smells. I want to be with Rob.

'Now now there's no need for tears,' says the woman. 'It will be time for your tablets soon.'

'I don't want any tablets. I'm not ill.'

'The woman smiles and shakes her head. 'You are my dear,' she says. 'That's why you are here in hospital.'

'I want to go home!' I yell. 'I'm going to Hollywood. I've no need to be here in some strange hospital.'

The woman laughs. 'You're in the right place,' she says.

A dark haired woman with a hard face and a burly looking man walk into the room pushing a strange looking cabinet on wheels.

'We've got a right one here,' says the woman. 'Seems to think she's something special.'

The man unlocks the cabinet and opens it. He looks like a gorilla.

'What's she down for?' asks the woman.

'Dunno, what's her name?'

Lorraine Tranmer.

'Let me see.' The man reads out from a piece of card.

'Just the usual knock out drops, largactil and Valium.'

'Well they should calm her down.'

The woman walks over to me with a small plastic cup containing four tablets.

'Take these, there's a good lass,' he says.

Don't take them, this is a bad place, says the voice inside my head.

I shake my head, keeping my mouth firmly closed.

'Come on,' says the man, 'I haven't got all day. Take your medication.'

They want to poison you because you're a bad person.

'No!' I scream. 'I don't need any tablets, let me go home. I don't need to be here, I'm not bad!' I run out of the room and pass the man who was sitting crying. He looks at me and his tears turn to hysterical laughter.

Suddenly a hand grabs my shoulder. I turn around. The man who was trying to give me the poison is accompanied by the two women.

They've got you now. They hate you, they want you dead.

They wrestle me to the ground and then sit on me.

'You had better calm yourself down,' says one of them.

They've got her now.

The voices in my head break into laughter.

'**They've got her now, they've got her now** ' *they* chant.

I lie there petrified, afraid to move a muscle.

'Are you going to come and take your tablets now?'

I nod my head timidly.

They stand up and I follow them back to the medicine trolley.

One of the women looks at me with distaste as once again she hands me the small plastic cup containing two white and two blue tablets. I place them in my mouth.

Is she going to swallow them?

She will surly perish if she does.

I turn around and spit the tablets into my hand.

'I saw that,' says the tablet keeper. 'Okay, have it your way, don't take them,' she says, shaking her head. ' But don't think I've forgotten.'

Ignoring the woman I go and sit in the corner of the room by the window.

'Where is this place that they have brought me to? And what am I really doing here? My Mam says it's a place of rest, but how can I rest here with all these strange people, people that sit staring with vacant glassy expressions and people that are trying to poison me?

Maybe they have brought me to the wrong place, or they could be trying to punish me for being bad and this place is a sort of prison, where people are held against their will.

The tablet keeper walks up to me. 'Would you come with me?' she says. 'I'm going to show you around the place.' I follow her upstairs and we enter a room which has beds on either side and a small table in the middle 'This is the dormitory,' she says. She stops and points to a bed halfway down the long room. 'This is where you will sleep,' she says. 'This room is out of bounds during the day.' She take me back down the stairs. 'This here is the recreation room,' she says as we enter another room.

I look around. A lady sits knitting and six or seven people are sitting around a table. They are not really doing anything. In the corner of the room sits a man of about Rob's age. He is in a wheelchair. Strange noises are coming from his mouth and saliva drips down his chin. He looks sad and my heart goes out to him. I leave my seat and go and stand by his side. 'Would you like me to sing to you?' I say, 'I can sing really well.'
The man doesn't say anything but the expression on his face changes and it looks like he's smiling at me. I rock his chair backwards and forwards and begin to sing.

'Will you shut up? I can't be doing with listening to this crap.'
I ignore the comment from the man sitting at the table and carry on singing.

The man at the table glares at me. 'You can't sing so just shut the fuck up!' he shouts.
Annoyed I turn around and face him. 'Do you know who I am?' I ask.
The man shrugs his shoulders, perplexed.
'I'm going to make it to the big time. I'm famous. Very soon my name will be on everyone's lips and as soon as I have had a rest I'm going on tour.'
I parade up and down the room singing and clapping as loudly as I can.
As the song comes to an end I drop a curtsey to my audience.
A woman laughs. 'Oh my god,' she says, 'she's away with the fairies.'
'Do you know where you are?'
I ignore the man sitting at the table.
'You are here with the rest of us in the bloody nut house and you ain't going no place.'
The man then gets up and leaves the room.

'Take no notice of him love, you're just in hospital,' says the woman.

'Hospital? I don't need to be here, I'm going on my tour, I'm…'

'You do love, you're just not well right now, got your pretty head full of fancy notions, you're just going to stay here until you're better and then go home again.'

'No, you're wrong, you're trying to fool me. I'm a brilliant singer, listen to me, just listen to me sing.' I then break into song and dance around the room.

An old woman puts her hands over her ears.

The man and woman who tried to give me poison walk over to me. 'Would you like to come this way?' they shout, trying to be heard above the noise that is coming from my mouth. 'There's someone in the office to see you.'

'It could be your agent,' smiles the man.

'I told you so,' I say to my 'audience.' 'It's my agent, I told you I was going to hit the big time.' Full of excitement and my own importance I eagerly follow the man and women into the office.

As soon as I walk into the office someone grabs hold of me. I see the shiny silver needle before my pants are pulled down and it is injected in my backside. I scream at the pain and tears of indignation run down my cheeks.

'You shouldn't have refused medication,' says the woman, 'so we had to give it to you the hard way.'

'You bastards!' I shout. 'Wait while I tell my agent.'

'There is no agent. You're sick and you're staying with us.'

'And who the hell are you, who do you think you are?' I scream

'We're the hospital staff and it would pay you to do as you are told in future.'

I walk away confused, wondering why I was brought to this strange place and thinking there must have been some kind of mistake.

You're done for now, chitter the voices inside my head.

You are theirs now.

The poison is in your veins it may even kill you.

I sit in my chair and feel the sweat running down my back as I await my fate.

Chapter 36

The next few days pass by in a haze. I have endured more injections which I believe is my punishment for deceiving my mother. Rob, my mother and an aunt and uncle I haven't seen in a long time came to see me this morning. I cried into Rob's arms when he left because I didn't want him to leave. My Mam says that I must stay here until I'm better. She says that I've had a nervous breakdown and that the voices in my head are not real, just like the strange thoughts I have. She tells me that they are all part of the illness and that I should ignore them. I don't believe her. I feel that she is like all the rest, the so called nursing staff and the doctors are all trying to hoodwink me.

I strongly believe that before I go on my tour I must stay here as a sort of test to see what sort of person I am and that the other people that sit in the day room or shuffle around the grounds are the unfortunate ones, the ones that have failed the test and have to stay here in this awful place. The man in the wheelchair's name is Alex. He has just been fed his dinner and has gravy running down his chin. I take a tissue and walk up to him and gently wipe his chin clean. I look into his vacant eyes and smile but he doesn't return my smile. Slowly I begin to rock him back and forth in his chair. At the same time I hum a little tune. This seems to comfort him as he closes his eyes and appears to go to sleep.

I slowly push him in his wheelchair to the quiet room so that he can get some peace and have a nice sleep. The room is empty as usual.

I push his chair into the corner of the room and pace his blanket around his knees.

Just as I'm about to leave the door opens abruptly and two men enter the room. They walk up to Alex.

'Don't wake him, he's just having a little rest' I say.

One of the men shakes his head. 'We can't have him sleeping during the day, he won't sleep tonight.'

The other member of staff laughs. 'I know what wakes him up,' he says.

He then takes the cover from Alex's knees, undoes his trousers and puts his hand down them.

Alex's eyes flick open.

'He likes that,' laughs the other member of staff. He then turns to me. 'Why don't you have a go?' he says. 'You are his little girlfriend.'

I feel my cheeks flame, as the bile rises up from my stomach.

Strange noises are coming from Alex's mouth.

I look away quickly.

'Go on, have a go, he likes you.'

I feel myself retching.

'Have a go.'

With my hand over my mouth I run from the room and run into the toilets where I immediately throw up over the chipped green tiles.

After that incident I stay away from poor Alex.

'I don't like it here,' I say to my Mam. 'I want to go home.'

My Mam looks up. She has tears in her eyes.

'As soon as you're well enough you can,' she says.

'Am I sick?' I ask.

'You are love. You have had some sort of breakdown.'

'My agent should be here any day now and then I will get away from this place and start my tour.'

My Mam sighs. 'You have to stop talking rubbish like that love,' she says, 'otherwise you will never get out of here.'

'What do you mean, rubbish?'

'You must get all these strange thoughts out of your mind and try to think clearly. Think of sensible things like getting well again, going back to work, seeing your friends and having a nice normal life.'

'But the voices, they tell me that…'

'The voices are all in your head Lorraine,' cuts in my Mam. 'Like I try to keep telling you, it's just your mind playing tricks with you.' My Mam walks over to me and places her arm around my shoulders. 'Try and get well love. We all miss you, and our little David and Michael keep asking when you are coming home.' I look up. My mam has tears in her eyes.

'But I'm not poorly am I?' I say.

My Mam kisses me on the forehead and holds me to her and I feel like a little child again. The bell then rings and I know it's time for my Mam to go home.

'I'll see you tomorrow.' I watch as my Mam walks slowly to the end of the room and out of the door. I brush away the tears that are spilling down my cheeks.

An old man sitting nearby overheard the conversation between myself and my Mam. He looks on and smiles sympathetically. 'Don't get upset little lass,' he says.

'Just concentrate on getting well, then you can go home with your Mammy, just remember what she told you.' The old man half smiles and points to his head. 'It's all in the mind lass,' he says, almost to himself.

'Ive been in this hospital for two years now and I've met a lot of people with strange ideas, just like you' says a middle aged woman.

'Hospital? Is this place really a hospital?' I ask.

'Yes it is, so don't go taking any notice of anyone saying it's a nut house. It's just a hospital like any other and what has happened to you can happen to anyone.'

Chapter 37

'Come on, get out of that bed, it's high time you were getting up.'
The damp bed sheets cling to me as I struggle to a sitting position.
In the back ground I can hear a whistle beeing blown and the sound of people cheering.
A matronly looking woman looks down at me. I read the badge attached to her jumper. It says STAFF NURSE SHIELDS.
'Come on, it's high time you were up,' she tuts. 'Fancy staying in bed on a lovely day like this. Everyone else is out in the fields. It's sports day, come on now, the doctor likes everyone to join in and the fresh air will do you the world of good.'
Hesitantly I climb out of bed. Nurse Shields pulls back my blankets and wrinkles her nose in distaste. She looks in my locker at the side of my bed. She takes my toilet bag and my towel. 'You need a shower,' she says. I stand in my wet nightdress. Sister Shields tuts impatiently. 'Come on then, let's take you to the bathroom.'

I stand under the shower cringing as the tepid water splashes on my body. Sister Sheilds hands me the bock of unscented soap. 'Make sure you wash yourself all over now,' she says.

I'm showered, dried and dressed in my underwear. Nurse Shield's hands me a pair of blue shorts and a faded pink T-shirt.
'I want you dressed and downstairs as soon as possible,' she says.
'Then you can have your breakfast and go and join the others on the field.'
The shorts are far to big for me and reach way passed my knees. I feel stupid and hope that today isn't the day my agent decides to come.
There's lots of activity going on in the large sports field.
The late summer sun is warm on my back and I have a horrible feeling in the pit of my stomach. I stand at the edge of the field with the other contestants waiting for the whistle to be blown and the race to start.
I look around at the many spectators watching and I feel like a goldfish in a bowl.
'They love to watch us loonies run,' says a man standing by my side.
The sharp shrill sound of the whistle fills my ear drums and the race

starts.   As I run my shorts fall down, reaching my ankles. I feel my cheeks flame as I stop and quickly pull them up. I can hear people laughing at me and tears of humiliation roll down my cheeks as I stumble last to the finishing line.

Lowering my head, I wander off the field.

Chapter 38

'Why don't you take the tablets my dear?' says the doctor. 'It can't be very pleasant for you having to have injections in your bottom all the time. It will be much easier for everyone if you agree to take your medication orally.'
I fidget in my seat.
The doctor stares at me from behind his desk. 'We are only trying to make you well, and the quicker you get well the quicker you can go home' The doctor stares at me over the top of his glasses. 'You do want to go home, don't you?' he asks.
I nod my head slowly.
'Well, you have a long way to go yet, but soon there may be a bed for you in the adolescents' ward. It will be better for you in there, and if you take your tablets your next step could be getting discharged.'
I stare out of the window. An ambulance pulls to a stop outside the main building.
'Am I sick?' I ask the doctor
'Yes you are, but if you take the tablets and try to relax you will start to feel a bit better.'
The doctor smiles and writes something down in the file in front of him. He then looks up. 'I'll have a little chat with you again in a few days time' he says looking up. 'You can go back to your ward now.'

The long days pass. I agree to take the tablets because I know they will give me the injections anyway, and I suppose taking the tablets is better then the painful numb feeling I get in my backside and the top of my leg each time I have an injection.

I sit in the day room listening to the radio. Just as I'm about to drop off to sleep Nurse Sheilds walks into the room. 'Lorraine, you have a visitor,' she says. I look up and my heart almost skips a beat as Rob smiles at me. Nurse Shields shakes her head and frowns as she walks out of the room.
He takes me in his arms and plants a soft kiss on my forehead.
'Are you feeling any better love?' he asks.
I shrug my shoulders. As I look around me an old lady sits rocking back and forth in her chair. 'I dunno,' I mutter, 'I just want to get

out of here. It doesn't seem like my agent's ever going to come.'

'Do you fancy a nice walk in the grounds?' asks Rob, changing the subject.

I nod my head eagerly and together we leave the ward.

It's a lovely day. The birds are singing and the scent from the flowers fills my nostrils.

Rob takes my hand. He towers above me and I feel safe and protected as I walk by his side. 'Do you want to play a sort of game?' he asks.

'Game. What game?'

'Well let's pretend,' says Rob, 'that this is Devil's Island and we have to find our way off it.'

'Okay, that sounds like a real good game.'

We cut through the patients' garden and enter a field. Laughing, we climb over the gate.

'This field leads to the road,' laughs Rob looking down at me. 'Don't worry, we'll soon be out of this place.'

Rob puts his arm around me and kisses me softly on the lips. 'This is no place for a young lass like you' he says as he holds me in his arms. He then looks furtively around him; the field is empty. The hospital is well behind us as we reach the road. Opposite the field stands a bus stop. We cross the road. 'Don't worry, we'll soon be far away from here,' he says as we make for the bus stop.

Presently the bus arrives. Smiling with relief, we climb on board and make for the back seat.

'We made it,' I say as I snuggle up in Rob's arms. 'We made it off the island.'

Chapter 39

'Where to?' says the conductor.

'Station please,' Rob fumbles in his pocket and brings out a small handful of change.

The conductor seems to look me up and down whilst Rob pays the fares.

I look away quickly, feeling sure that he knows me. Without saying a word he clips our tickets and hands them to Rob.

The bus speeds along the road. I sit with my head leant on Rob's shoulder, wondering if anyone at the hospital had noticed that I had escaped.

Rob smiles at me. 'You okay?' he asks.

I look into his eyes and nod my head like an obedient puppy dog.

'Good,' says Rob.

As the bus stops at various stops letting people off and on, I bury my head in Rob's shoulder so as not to be recognized.

Presently we reach the centre of town.

'It's nearly time to get off,' says Rob, giving me a gentle nudge as he thinks I'd fallen asleep.

We get off the bus.

Rob takes my hand and together we leave the station.

'I'll take you to my mate's flat,' says Rob. 'He says I can stay there whenever I want. He's all right is Mark and his girlfriend Julie will look after you. It will be better then you having to stay in that bloody nut house with all those strange people.'

'But my agent,' I say, 'how will he know where I am?'

Rob glares at me. 'Look here,' he says, 'stop talking crap. There is no agent so try to get it out of your mind and when you get to the flat don't go on about agents and things or tell anyone you have just broken out of the nut house.' Rob shakes his head and for the first I can see anger in his eyes.

'It's just you and me now babe,' he says.

'Are we going to get married then?'

Rob smiles and his face softens. 'Of course we are Lorraine,' he mutters.

We walk down a long street, and stop outside a black and white house.

'Here we are,' says Rob. 'Me mate and his bird live in the top flat.'

Rob then throws a small pebble up to the window.

I hear someone rolling the window down.

'It's only me,' says Rob.

'Come on up mate!" says a man as he throws down a key. We enter the hallway. It's dirty and stinks of neglect. As we go up the stairs a baby cries and a woman shouts.

Presently we reach the top and Rob unlocks the door to number twenty two.

We enter a small room which has another room just off it.

A blonde haired woman walks out of the other room still wearing her dressing gown.

'Hiya Julie, you just got up?' says Rob.

The woman smiles and nods her head.

A man wearing a pair of filthy jeans and a T-shirt looks my way.

'Who's this then Rob?' he says. 'I didn't know you were into cradle snatching.'

'This is Lorraine my new bird and...' Rob hesitates, 'she's almost eighteen.'

I feel my face burning and I hope I don't give the game away.

'Yeah, pull the other one,' says the man. 'She only looks about fourteen to me.'

'Do you think you can put us up for a few days Mark?' asks Rob, ignoring his comment.

'You'll have to kip on the floor,' says Mark.

'That will be fine Mark.'

Julie smiles. 'Wanna a cup of tea love?' she asks.

I nod my head gratefully.

'Hey, haven't you got a tongue in your head?' laughs Julie as she takes the kettle and walks over to the small sink in the corner of the room.

'She's a bit shy,' says Rob, coming to my defence.

'Well she need not be shy with me.' Julie fills the kettle and places it on to the hob.

'You take sugar and milk?' she asks.

'One sugar please.'

'Oh well you have got a voice then.'

I look around the room. It doesn't contain much furniture, just a grubby three seat sofa and a table in the corner. The floor is covered in dull grey canvas with a faded almost threadbare rug lying in the centre. Cackling music plays from an ancient looking wireless standing beneath the window. A dirty chipped sink and cupboard stand next to a small stove. An unlit gas fire is positioned below the dusty mantelpiece which contains a clock and a small framed photograph of Julie and Mark.

Clouds of dust rise in the damp atmosphere and there is a sort of musky smell about the place which makes me think of unwashed bodies.

'Sit yourself down,' says Julie, pointing to the sofa.

I sit down. The sofa feels hard and lumpy.

'How long are you planning on staying?' says Mark.

'Oh, we just need to stay a few days until we find our own place.'

'We?' said Mark, looking puzzled.

'Yeah, me and Lorraine.'

'Does her mother know she's out?' asks Julie with a sarcastic edge to her voice.

'Yeah, of course,' said Rob, 'I told you, she's nearly eighteen.'

'She'd better not be a runaway,' said Mark, 'I can't be doing with the coppers coming round here nosing about.'

Rob sighs. 'No, everything's above board,' he says.

'As long as it is,' said Mark.

Julie smiles. 'Stay as long as you need to,' she says. 'It will be nice having anther female around the place.' She hands me my cup of tea and I sit back on the sofa and drink it gratefully, for up until then my mouth felt so parched. I was told in the hospital this was a side effect of the tablets. 'Well,' I think to myself, 'there will be no more tablets now.'

We sit in the flat listening to the radio. My stomach growls. I realize that I haven't eaten all day. I don't like to tell anyone how hungry I feel. I look at the clock on the mantelpiece. It's eleven thirty. I yawn, for I've been up since six that morning and it has been a long and eventful day for me.

Eventually and much to my relief Mark and Julie go to the bedroom, leaving Rob and me sitting on the sofa. The sofa is too small for us both to sleep on so we make a bed on the floor. Having undressed we lie in the dark Rob puts his arm around me and begins to smother my face with kisses. I kiss him back. He lies on top of me. His body feels heavy against mine and the floorboards feel hard on my back whilst he roughly takes me.

Rob turns away as soon as it's over.

'You didn't put up much of a struggle, did you?' he spits almost

disappointedly. 'And I could tell you weren't a virgin.'
I think of Danny, my first love, and how different he'd been to Rob
and my eyes fill with tears.
'I don't respect you any more, you're nothing but a crazy little slut.'
The next morning Rob is in a different mood. He brings me a cup of
tea to bed as though last night had never happened.
'I want to go home,' I say.
'Don't be stupid. If you do your Mam will send you back to the
fucking loony bin.'
'But my agent, he won't know where I am.'
Rob's eyes blaze with anger. 'I've told you!' he says, 'I've told you
not to talk crap like that, how many fucking times do I have to tell
you there is no bloody agent!'
'There is, the voices told me so.'
'What fucking voices?'
'The voices in my head.'
Rob looks at me with disdain. 'You're one crazy little chick' is all he
says.

Chapter 40

'For Christ's sake, you've pissed all over me! I'm soaking wet through. Get up and go to toilet!'

I sit bolt upright in our make shift bed on the floor. Julie's spare blankets feel damp and cold to my skin. Hesitantly I stand up. The room is in semi darkness, and I hear the birds singing the morning chorus as I make my way along the landing.

Trembling I reach the small room on the left which contains the toilet and a small dirty sink. I sit on the toilet for some time, afraid and overcome with embarrassment. My head aches and my stomach growls, complaining of hunger. Suddenly I hear a knock on the door.

'Hurry up in there will you, I'm dying for a piss!' shouts a woman's voice. I slowly turn the handle of the door and step out and I'm greeted with the women from the flat downstairs who shares the toilet.

'Bloody hell, she's stark naked,' she says to herself as I walk by her, 'must be on drugs or something.'

I stand by the door. Rob is sitting on the sofa. 'Julie isn't going to be to happy about the state of her blankets; you've pissed them right through,' he says. 'That's twice you've done that in the week we've been here.'

My legs seem to wobble as I walk across the room. Without warning the floor comes up to meet me and I welcome the blackness.

'Wake up love, wake up.'

I open my eyes and see Rob's face above mine. 'That's it, take it easy.'

'You feeling better now?' asks Julie. 'Rob told me you had a sort of a fit, you've been out of it for the past hour.'

Tears rain down my face. 'I want my Mam,' I mutter.

'Oh Rob, she's only a baby, I think it will be for the best if you take her home.'

'I can't,' says Rob 'I sort of love her. Besides, there will be trouble if I do take her home.'

Julie sighs. 'How old did you say she was?'

'Rob puts his head down. 'She's fifteen,' he says.

'I knew it,' says Mark, 'she is a runaway, ain't she?'

Rob nods his head slowly.

'The poor little bugger needs a doctor. She's sick, passing out like that, it just isn't normal, and she talks to herself as well, I've heard her,' says Julie.

'Yeah, she's a strange one all right, look, she's just staring into space.

'I want to go home,' I mutter.

'It's okay love,' says Mark, giving Rob a dirty look. 'We'll see you get home safe and sound.'

We walk to the town centre then on to the bus station.

Rob gives me my bus fare and Julie and Mark look away whilst Rob holds me in his arms and kisses me. He has tears in his eyes. 'I'll see you again one day,' is all he says before putting me on the number seventy six bus. It's a new pay as you enter bus. I give the driver the five pence bus fare. 'Half to Hedon' I stutter. The driver smiles and gives me my ticket.

As the bus pulls out of the station I look out of the window and wave to Rob Julie and Mark. They look up and wave back.

I sit back in my seat. A man and woman sit opposite me. The woman mutters something to the man and they both stare at me. I feel certain that they both know everything about me, so I lower my head.

Presently a man dressed in a blue uniform gets on the bus. My heart sinks. I think it's a policeman who's come to take me back to the hospital. He walks up the aisle and stops at my seat cold sweat runs down my back..

'Can I see your ticket please,' he asks. With relief I realise he's an inspector.

I show him my ticket and he nods his head and walks on.

The bus pulls up at every stop. I keep my head low as other passengers board the bus.

The smell from the factories tells me that the bus has reached Hedon road. Raising my head I quickly glance out of the window. We pass the hospital where I'd been born. A sadness tightens my heart as I remember the time when I'd sat in that handcart, excited at the prospect of a new start. I recall the proud look on my dad's face as he'd pulled the handcart into his home town.

Finally we reach Hedon and my stomach turns in a knot. The bus reaches my stop. Hesitantly I stand up and make my way to the

front of the bus. The driver shoots me a suspicious look as I step off
the platform.

I run down Church Lane as fast as my legs can carry me and stop
outside number twenty four. Grahame is in the garden. He looks at
me as though he has seen a ghost.
'Mam, Mam!' he shouts. 'Our Lorraine's come home!'
My Mam comes out of the house and runs towards me.
'Oh, where have you been love?' she says, relief showing clearly on
her worried lined face. Without waiting for an answer she takes me
in her arms and together we walk into the house. My cousin and her
boyfriend look at me as though unable to believe their eyes. 'Oh,
thank God you're home,' says Geoff, my cousin's boyfriend. 'I've
looked all over Hull for you, where the Hell have you been?'
A woman named Ann who lives just a few doors down is sitting on
the sofa.
'If you only knew what you've put your poor mother through,' she
says, shaking her head. She picks up the coffee cup by her side and
sips it. 'Fancy running away like that, you've nearly driven your
mother round the bend as well...'
'Do you mind leaving,' says my Mam. 'It's been good of you to
come and sit with me but I need to talk to Lorraine right now.'
'Okay Jean, I understand,' says Ann, who after shooting me a cross
look leaves the room.
'You'd better ring the police and The Daily Mail up Auntie Jean,'
said Sue, my cousin, 'and let them know she's home.'
Grahame picks up a photo of me. 'That was going in tomorrow's
paper' he says. 'The police have been and everything.'
I burst into tears. 'Don't let them send me back to that place Mam,
please,' I say in between sobs.
'Don't worry love, I don't intend to,' says my Mam. 'You're staying
here with me, at least then I know you're safe.'
'And then my agent will know where I am,' I say, almost to myself.
My Mam looks at me through her tears and sighs.

Chapter 41

The policewoman looks at me long and hard. 'Now Lorraine,' she says at length, 'would you like to tell me where you have been?'
'It was him,that Rob, he took her out of the hospital. The poor little bugger didn't know what was going on' says my mam.
'Let Lorraine answer for herself' says the policewoman.
'But she's very ill, she's in no fit state to speak to you, can't you see she's afraid? She's gone as white as a bottle of milk.'
I bite down hard on my bottom lip. My mouth feels dry and I can feel my heart beating madly beneath my T-shirt. There is a silence.
'Answer the lady Lorraine love,' coaxes my Mam. 'Tell her what you told me.'
'We played a game,' I said slowly.
'A game?'
'We were on Devil's Island and we escaped,' I mutter.
'I thought she was in a safe place,' says my Mam.
The policewoman writes something down..
I burst into tears. 'Please don't take me back.'
'Back where?' says the policewoman.
'To that place. I don't want to go back there ever.'
'You mean the hospital?'
I nod my head.
'Don't worry love,' says my Mam, 'you're staying here with me, where I know you're safe.'
The police women finishes taking my statement and leaves.
After that is the visit to the doctor's. He agrees with my Mam that it will be in my best interests if I stay at home. He writes me a prescription for some Valium and another tablet with a funny sounding name which sounds something like largactil. He tells my Mam that these will take away my strange thoughts and get rid of the voices. And the Valium will keep me calm. However, I still have to see the psychiatrist as an outpatient.
Filled with relief at the thought of not having to return to the hospital, I shake the doctor by the hand and my Mam and I leave the surgery.
Because it was disclosed during the interview with the police that I wasn't a virgin when Rob took me away they decide not to prosecute him. However, Rob is wanted on other charges.

****

As the weeks pass the tablets begin to take effect and the voices gradually disappear.

I also stop believing in what they said to me and start to accept the fact that I had been very ill.   I stop waiting for 'my agent,' and slowly begin to realise that it was just a delusion which was a part of the illness.

One doctor tells my Mam that I was going through a teenage crisis and another one said that I was suffering a schizophrenic attack, so it's difficult to say what it really was.

I feel I owe my Mam so much because if it wasn't for her care I would most likely still be in that hospital.

I sit with my Mam on the sofa. We have been having a talk.

'I'm so glad you're better love,' she says. 'Now all we need to do is build you up.'

I nod my head in agreement because physically I feel quite weak and only weigh five and a half stone wet through.

'If there is ever anything bothering you I want you to tell me about it,' says my Mam.

'There used to be,' I said.

'What was it?'

'I used to think that no one really cared about me and that I was dirty.'

'But Lorraine love, me and your dad have always cared about you.'

'I know you do now Mam.'

'What made you think such a thing, was it something I did, something I said?'

'Do you remember that Uncle Ralph?'

My Mam's face turns pale at the mention of his name. 'I didn't think you remembered him' she says.

'I know it was a long time ago Mam, but I never forgot him and what he did... And because nothing was ever done about it I just thought you didn't care and...'

I trail off.

'We tried Lorraine, we told the copper who was on the beat at that time and he more or less advised us what to do. He felt that it would be a traumatic experience for you having to go through the courts at such a young age. So he told us to take the law in our own hands...'

'And did you?'

'Yes your dad well, he gave him a good hiding in that passage, and well, that was that.

We never spoke about it to you. We were hoping you would forget all about it.'

My Mam sighs deeply. 'But to think you've carried it on your little shoulders all these years.   Maybe we should have ignored that copper's advice and taken it to the courts, but we just did what we thought was for the best at the time.'

'Never mind Mam, at least now I know you did care about me.'

'There's no wonder you had a breakdown though, keeping that bottled up in your head all that time.'

'It might have happened anyway.'

'We'll never know that, will we Lorraine?'

'Well, let's not talk about it any more today. I'm okay now Mam and that's the main thing.'My Mam kisses me on the forehead. 'Don't ever keep anything bottled up inside you again will you love?' she says.

'No Mam, I'll try not to.'

Later that night I lie awake in bed listening to the rain pattering on the windows.

'Its all out in the open now,' I tell myself, feeling a huge weight has been taken from my mind. Hopefully everything could be all right now...

Ladybird Ladybird Fly away Home

Lorraine Ellis

Some names in this book have been changed

Lorraine Ellis

Acknowledgements

I would like to thank my family and also my friend Liz Marritt for their encouragement and support.

And a big thanks to my daughter Lucy Ellis for the drawing on the front cover.

Lorraine Ellis

Chapter 1

You're a bad Mother your daughter's in danger and all you do is lie in that stinking bed.
I sit up and look around me there is no one in the bedroom I glance at the clock it's Six thirty, Pete has left for work I am alone.
You're wicked.
I put my head in my arms but it doesn't drown out the voices.
Your Daughter's in great peril and yet you do nothing.
You're evil.
Convinced now, I quickly get out of bed.
I pass Samantha and Cheryl's bedroom they're both sleeping soundly.
I then glance in Lucy's room and to my horror her bed is empty.
She's in danger, she's in danger.

My heart beating rapidly and the sweat running down my back I take the stairs two at a time.
I dress quickly and run out the house the cold air hits me for all I'm wearing is a thin cotton skirt and T-shirt.
I run as fast as I can to my mam's house, frantically   I burst into the living room.
Michelle, my brother's wife sits on the sofa drinking a cup of tea.
'What's wrong love?' asks my mam.
'It's Lucy my baby, she's in danger.'
'Don't be daft Lorraine she's fast asleep upstairs in bed cosy and warm don't you remember she stayed here the night last night.'
I have no memory of this so I eye her suspiciously.
Pay no heed to what she says she's part of the plan.
My dad walks into the room,
'Hiya love, you're here early, you feeling any better, you didn't look well at all yesterday don't you remember fainting in the kitchen.'
Don't listen to him he's trying to fool you.
'I've come to get Lucy, she's coming home with me now.'
'Come back in a couple of hours, the bairns fast asleep it's a shame to disturb her go home and get some rest yourself you look bloody terrible.'

My Dad looks around the room, 'Anyway where's the other two?'

It's then I realise that in my panic I'd left Sammy and Cheryl alone in the house.'

'Look, I'll come back with you,' said my Mam. 'We'll have a cup of tea and a chat and then we'll perhaps get the doctor out to you because you're just not yourself love.'

Don't trust her! Shout the voices

I run to the door,' look after my Lucy,' I scream at Michelle as I run out into the street.

Ladybird Ladybird fly away home,
Your house is on fire and your children are dead.

The voices sing inside my head as I run.

I turn around to discover my Mam is running after me.

'You're in hurry this morning' says the milkman with a puzzled expression on his face.

I reach my House. As soon as I get in I go up the stairs to my relief I discover my kids are still in their beds fast asleep, oblivious to everything.

By the time I return down the stairs my Mam has entered my house and is filling the kettle at the sink.

'Sit down and relax love,' she says, 'I think you're having a breakdown I know the signs all too well.'

Make her go away.

She's not to be trusted.

I snatch the kettle out of her hands water slops on to the blue lino.

'Leave me alone! Please just get out of my house.'

'But love, I'm here to help you.'

'No you're not, get out now!'

'I'm not leaving you in this state , you're sick again,' I follow my Mam into the living room, she sits on the sofa. 'Don't you remember that breakdown you had when you were fifteen _____well I think you're having another one love.' My mam wipes away a tear..

Don't listen to her for she cries crocodile tears.

I run out of the door and go to a neighbour's house a few doors away.

'I need to use your phone,' I say quickly.

Seeing the look of panic on my face Jane hands me the receiver and I quickly dial the numbers nine, nine, nine.

'Police fire or ambulance,' says the operator.

'Police it's urgent.'

'Speak slowly,' said the operator.

'Will you come and get my Mother out of my house!' I shout.

I then give my address and slam the receiver back in its cradle.

Jane looks on perplexed.

'What's going on Lorraine?' she says.

'It's my Mother she won't leave and she's not to be trusted she's all a part of the plan.'

'Don't be daft Lorraine,' says Jane 'you think the world of your Mam, I mean you go and see her every single day, do you want to sit down and tell me what's wrong?.'

'I just want to be safe,' I shout as I run up her stairs.

I enter a bedroom, it smells of honeysuckle and I think back to when I was a child. I sit by her bed a secure feeling washes over me.

Jane comes into the room with a concerned look on her face.

'Can I stay here a while?' I ask.

'If you want Lorraine,' she says puzzled.

I kneel by the side of the bed with all sorts of thoughts running around my head.

You must atone for your sins,' says the voices.

I have never been a religious person but I lock my hands in prayer and rock myself backwards and forwards.

After some time Jane slowly opens the door.

'The police are downstairs Lorraine they just need to talk with you.'

Relieved now, I stand up, my knees ache and my head throbs.

The policeman looks me up and down.

'You can go back home now,' he says 'your Mother's gone.'

'Am I safe?'

'Yes your fine.' The policeman half smiles and looks at Jane as together they walk towards the front door. I stay where I am in the living room listening to the dull murmur if their voices. It's difficult to make out what they discussing but I hear Jane saying something about 'the doctor's on his way,' and I wonder who's been taken ill. I sit on Jane's sofa with jumbled up thoughts running around my head.

'Now don't worry about anything,' says Jane coming into the room 'the girls have been taken to school and they're alright.'

'My babies, I'd left them alone in that house.'

'You were just down the road,' says Jane, 'don't worry about the kids, it's yourself you want to be worried about.'

She's a bad mother,

Evil, wicked.

And she's going to Hell.

'Let me make you a cup of tea.'

'Am I wicked?'

'No you're a good lass, you're just not yourself right now.'

'But can't you hear what they're saying about me?'

'What who's saying?'

'The voices, the voices!'

Jane takes my hand, 'there's no one here but us Lorraine,' she says.

'You might hear them soon,' I say

'I don't know what you're talking about,'

I follow Jane into the kitchen, 'it must be stress,' she mutters to herself.

I watch as the steam from the kettle rises upwards.

She hates you really, hiss the voices

The tea made, Jane carries the cups into the living room.

I sit on the couch sipping my tea it tastes exceptionally sweet.

She wants to poison you.

With a lump in my throat I quickly place the cup by my side, I stand up to leave

'Stay with me a while,' says Jane.

'No, I got to go now,' I mutter.

'Just stay a little longer.'

Just as I'm about to leave, the living room door opens and my G.P briskly walks into the room.

'Oh doctor,' says Jane, 'Lorraine isn't too well today.

'Would you like to tell me what's bothering you,' Doctor Harris smiles at me.

I pace up and down the living room saying nothing.

'Come and sit down.' Doctor Harris guides me to the sofa.

'I think her nerves are bad or something,' says Jane, who then in a low voice goes on to tell Doctor Harris the events of the morning.

'I think she may be having panic attacks,' says the doctor opening his bag from where he takes out a small bottle. He hands me two tablets.

Jane fetches a small glass of water,

'There are just a mild sedative but they should help calm you down.'

I look at the two blue tablets in my hand.

'Come on now take them,' says the doctor firmly.

Gingerly, I place them in my mouth and swallow them. I then sit back on the sofa waiting...... waiting for death.

'That's better, just relax,' the doctor picks up his bag and is gone in a breeze.

Chapter 2

My head feels numb as I slowly sit up.

'Feeling any better now Lorraine?' says Jane, 'you've been asleep ages.'

I place my hand on my heart and feel it beating.

'Am I dead?'

'No you've just had a sleep that's all; those tablets knocked you out for the count.'

I bite down hard on my bottom lip until I can taste blood.

'I'll take you back home,' says Jane. Pam's round at your house I told her your nerves are bad, she's going to sit with you until Pete comes home.'

She's bad, cackle the voices.

I turn to Jane, 'am I bad?' I ask.

'No you're not bad it's your nerves that are bad

My head feels fuzzy like it does when you have been sleeping for a really long time.

Jane fetches me a glass of water. Despite being very thirsty I quickly place it by my side.

'Come on,' says Jane 'I'll take you home.'

On legs that feel like jelly I walk towards the door.

'I'm alright,' I falter.

Jane stands on her step watching every move I make as I walk up her garden path.

'It's me Mam, it's me Mam!' shouts Lucy as soon as I enter the house.

Relieved to see that she's safe I hold her to me.

Sammy smiles from her chair in the corner she's watching the television.

I walk up to her and kiss her soft cheek.

Where you been Mammy?' says Cheryl

Bending down I pick up my five year old and hold her in my arms, tears run down my face.

I look around the room. Pam a close relative of ours walks in from the kitchen.

'The state of it in there,' she snaps 'you can't see the sink for the pots and there is dirty washing everywhere.

I hold Cheryl tighter to me.

Where's my Pete?.'
'He's at work you know he is, and put that child down you might frighten her.'
You're going to die soon, says a taunting voice inside my head.
I burst into sobs.
'He won't be home for a while so in the mean time I suggest you pull yourself together. I don't know what your neighbours are going to think,'
I sit in the arm chair with Cheryl on my knee. She looks up at me.
'What's matter mammy?' she asks.
'Oh your Mother's just being silly take no notice of her.'
'I want Pete,' I say in a voice that doesn't sound like mine.
Pam tuts disapprovingly. 'I think you should be thinking about getting his tea ready he'll have had an hard day on the building site, never mind having to come home to this pandemonium.' She clucks.
'Mammy I'm hungry,' says Cheryl.
Bad mother, bad mother.
Pam shoots me a disdainful look she walks into the kitchen and I hear cupboard doors. opening and slamming shut., 'Just a few tins of beans and hardly a crust of bread in the house.' I hear her mutter.
A strong feeling of guilt washes over me when I realise I haven't done any shopping today.
'Beans and blooming toast that's a fine meal to give a man after he's done an hard day's work,.'
Cheryl clambers off my knee and joins her sisters who are sitting on the living room floor watching the television.
My head throbs as the voices spit out their venom.
You're an utter disgrace.
Useless
A bitch.
Wicked,
The wickedest woman in the world.
She's been here before.
She's older than time.
She's the chosen one.

I hear a loud cry and it is sometime before I realise it is me that's crying. And as the .racking sobs engulf my body Doctor Harris enters the room.
'She's almost hysterical Doctor,' says Pam as she scurries about picking up toys.

'Mammy's crying,' says Cheryl.

'Go and play upstairs a bit that's good girls'

With troubled looks etched on their little faces my babies leave the living room. .

I can't get my breath, my head spins.

'Relax now Lorraine take some deep breaths,' says the doctor slowly his voice sounding like it's coming from a long way.'

She'll die soon.

She's the chosen one.

'I don't want to die,' I say in between sobs.

'You're not dying you're alright you're quite safe.'

My sobs reduce to a quiet whimper.

'That's it calm down,'

I hear the front door open and the familiar tread of Pete's boots as he walks up the hallway.

I breathe a sigh of relief.

'Mr Ellis have you any idea what's bothering your wife has anything happened to upset her recently?'

Pete shakes his head and there is a silence Pam hovers in the background.

'Am I the chosen one?' I ask.

Pete looks on a bit perplexed.

'You're saying some silly things Lorraine,' says the doctor.

'They tell me I'm the chosen one.'

'Who tells you this,'

'Them the voices didn't you hear them.

'Try and relax there's no one here but us and nothing bad is going to happen,.

Doctor Harris turns to Pete, 'I feel your wife is suffering from nervous exhaustion.' He nods his head as though agreeing with himself, Pete stares at the wall a thing he always does when he's troubled. There is a silence in the small room broken only by the sounds of the kids playing in their room above.

'Lorraine?' says Doctor Harris at length 'how would you feel about going somewhere for a little rest. It won't be for long, perhaps just a week or two until you feel a little better.'

I glance at Pete he looks sad and tired, it might be for the best love he says gently.'

Doctor Harris nods his head, 'I'll make the necessary arrangements,' he says before leaving the house.

Chapter 3

'Come this way love,' says the uniformed man as he guides me down the path'

I look ahead an ambulance is parked by our front gate and I wonder who's ill.

Turning around I see Pam and my girls standing on the step.

'Where's me mam going?' asks Lucy in a small voice.'

'She's just going on a little holiday,' says Pam.

I hear Sammy start to cry.

'Mammy poorly,' says Cheryl.

The front door closes abruptly.

Pete carries my case towards the waiting ambulance and it is then that I realise the ambulance is meant for me. The man helps me inside.

'I'll come and see you every day love,' says Pete as the doors closes.

The ambulance

We've got her now.

moves on

I sit bolt upright in my seat.

'Don't be afraid,' the ambulance man looks through me and it seems like he's looking inside my mind.

'There's nothing to worry about just sit back in your seat and we'll be there .before you know it.'

I lower my head feeling certain that the ambulance driver can read my every thought.

'Get out you're not coming in,' I tell me self 'get out of my head.

'You'll feel better soon, they'll   have you as right as ninepence in a few days.'

Don't look at him.

I close my eyes.

'That's it have a little rest.'

He hates you really.

Despite the fact that the ambulance man thinks I'm sleeping he tries to strike up a conversation with me. Keeping my eyes tightly closed I ignore him.

After what seems like an eternity   I feel the ambulance man pat me on the shoulder,' 'we're here love,' he says.

I look out the window.

The first thing I notice is a large Victorian building which stretches upwards towards the oppressive grey sky. The place seems to have a vague familiarity about it almost as though I'd seen it before perhaps in a dream
On the left and right of the drive are smaller buildings which look equally as old and forbidding as the main one.' The ambulance pulls to a stop outside one of them.
The doors are slid open and I'm led outside.
.

'This is Garton ward,' the ambulance man takes my case and leads me to the entrance. Hesitantly I step inside.
A tall dark haired woman walks up to us.
I've just brought the new admittance nurse,' says the ambulance man
I glance at the nurse. She doesn't look like a nurse for it appears that she's chewing gum and isn't even wearing a uniform.
The Ambulance man turns to me,' bye then love,' he says' and don't worry like I say you'll be as right as nine-pence in a few days,' he then turns and walks away.

******

I'm sitting in a small room opposite a desk. Behind the desk sits the nurse and to the side of her sits a man dressed in a grey suit.
The voices laugh and cackle.
She's bad, she's wicked she's no good.
'Leave me alone!' I shout, 'please just go away.
I place my hands over my head.
The nurse looks up, 'it's okay,' she says holding her pen in midair, 'no one is going to hurt you, you're quite safe. The doctor's just going to ask you a few questions
This is a bad place.
I feel my heart beating beneath my T-shirt.
'My name's Doctor Gregson,' says the man wearing the grey suit, 'would you like to tell me what yours is?'
I ignore him and try to look away avoiding his gaze but his eyes are fixed on me and he stares at me long and hard. 'Okay then can you tell me what day this is?'
This time I can't answer the doctor whether I want to or not because I've no idea what day it is as the last few have all seemed to have merged into one.'

'What's your date of birth?'

Saying nothing I manage to look away from the doctor but I can still feel his eyes burning into me. The clock on the wall ticks away as the doctor waits patiently for the answers to his questions.

'She's unresponsive today nurse so we'll try again tomorrow,' I hear the doctor say in a low voice.

We are then dismissed from the room.

'I'll show you around the ward,' says the nurse, we walk down the corridor I stare at the grey tiles and the stale smell of urine fills my nostrils. We enter a room where a group of people sit around a blaring television. .

I look around, a lady looks up from her knitting, 'Is that tea trolley coming soon! she shouts trying to make her voice heard above the noise coming from the television set. A man sits in a corner staring at nothing. The nurse walks up to the television set and turns down the volume 'this is the dayroom,' she says. We then walk out of the room down the corridor and up two flights of stairs. The nurse opens the door to a long room. A row of beds face each other the nurse stops at a bed about halfway down the room.

'This is the ladies dormitory and this is your bed,' she says. She then places my case on top of the locker by the bed. 'You can unpack now.'

I open my case and place my toilet bag, night wear, and change of clothes in the small locker.

'Is that all you've brought with you?' I nod my head.

'Never mind you can have some more clothes sent in and we have plenty that will fit you in the spare clothing cupboard.' The nurse looks at her watch, 'it's almost bedtime,' she says 'so I'll leave you here to unpack you may as well change into you nightgown and get into bed. Someone will be up soon with your medication.' The nurse turns away. I hear the clicking of her heels as she walks back up the dormitory and out of the door.

This is a bad place.

I sit up rigidly on the edge of the bed as a feeling of dread washes over me.

I think of Pete and the kids, and I wonder if I will ever see them again.

Tears of fear and sadness roll down my cheeks.

Presently the door opens and a woman comes into the dormitory. She stops by my bed and hands me a small plastic cup filled with water she then hands me two tablets.

'Take your medication,' she says. She stands watching whilst I hesitantly place the tablets in my mouth
'Good girl,' she says taking the cup from my hand.
I burst into tears.
'Don't get upset now, I know it's a bit strange at first but you'll soon get settled in.
I look at her through my tears she too is wearing casual clothes I look at the name badge pinned to her jumper it reads Margaret then in smaller letters underneath it says Staff Nurse. She walks to my locker and takes out my nightclothes, 'come on,' she says 'let's have you ready for bed, by the look of you a good night's sleep will do you good.'

'That's better,' she says pulling back the bed sheet.
I get into bed. She tucks the blanket around me and I feel like a child again.
'You'll feel better in a few days, she says, 'try to get some sleep the others will be up soon.'
I hear the jingling of keys as she walks away.

My eyelids feel heavy now and despite my anxiety I close them and let myself slowly drift away.

Chapter 4

I'm jolted awake to the sounds of someone snoring and a woman crying, then the laughter begins.

You're dead, cackles the voice inside my head.

Suddenly I'm standing by my locker I look on my bed and can see the form of someone lying there.

Your soul has left your body.

I run past the rows of beds.

You can't get away you're dead.

Startled by my own screams I run towards the door and I'm met by a heavily built woman 'Stop making such a din calm yourself down, you'll wake everyone else up.' She says.' I feel sharp finger nails dig into my flesh as she grabs my arm and drags me out of the dormitory door and down the stairs. She then takes me to a small room containing nothing but a bean bag. 'You can stay here and scream as loud as you want,' she then closes the door with a bang.

.I shudder as I remember a book I had once read which was written by a medium in the book the medium claimed that when you die you wake up in a sort of hospital.

I stand in the centre of the room with urine running down my legs. Petrified I pinch my flesh and wonder if I'm alive.

After some time the door opens, staff nurse Margaret walks in. 'Glad you've quietened yourself down,' she says,'come on I'll take you to the bathroom.   Holding my toilet bag and my change of clothes she ushers me out of the room.

The bathroom is cold and the water runs tepid from the large Victorian taps, Staff nurse Margaret stands and watches me whilst I get undressed. Quickly I step into the bath . I feel my cheeks flame as the nurse proceeds to wash my body she pulls out the plug.   I slowly stand up trying hard to cover my dignity.

'Oh don't worry I've seen it all before and you're no different to any other woman'.

The rough towel chafes my skin as I quickly dry myself.

Once dressed the nurse ushers me out of the door, down the stairs and into dinning room. 'As a rule you should be making your bed in the dormitory,' she says 'but perhaps it will be for the best if we wait while you're more settled.

A line of people are standing by a serving hatch. The nurse hands me a tray,
'wait in line with the rest of them.' she says.
I take my place and stand at the end of the line. An old woman turns around to face me. 'Was that you I heard screaming in the early hours of this morning my God you made enough noise to raise the dead. 'Were you having a nightmare or something?'
Shuddering I swallow back the saliva in my mouth.
I reach the front of the queue where a man wearing a plastic apron faces me from behind the serving hatch., 'What's it to be?' he asks 'Cereal, toast, sausage and egg, or all three?'
'Cereal please,' I mutter

My cornflakes are poured out into a plastic bowl. I then slowly carry my tray to a nearby table.
'You should have got yourself a cooked breakfast,' says the old woman, it's the only decent meal you ever get in this place'
The cereal tastes like cardboard in my mouth having managed to swallow just two spoonfuls I stand up and leave the table

I enter the main room where people are sitting in separate little groups, some of them chatting, some laughing, and some crying. But most of them aren't doing anything and just sit motionlessly or rock backwards and forwards with sad empty expressions etched on their lined faces.
'All things bright and beautiful all creatures great and small, all things wise and wonderful the lord God made them all,' sings a women' in a shrill bird like voice.
'What the fucking hell is beautiful in here,' grumbles a man in the corner.'
'Now Bob that isn't very nice,' the nurse sighs as she gives out the morning medication.

I pace up and down the room thinking of Pete and wonder what the kids are doing and how they are going to cope without me and most of all how I'm going to cope without them.
.'Lorraine go and sit yourself down,' says a nurse 'you've been walking up and down for the best part of an hour you'll wear yourself out.

The nurse takes my hands and like a child I'm led to sit down on a nearby armchair.

'This is Lorraine and she's come to stay for a while.'

'My names Nancy,' says a middle aged woman, 'how you feeling?'

'Am I dead?' I ask.

'No you're quite safe you're here with us.'

'Might as well be fucking dead than shut up in this bloody hole,' mutters a man.

'Watch your flaming Language Bob,' laughs Nancy .

'Aye okay Nance,' Bob takes his tobacco and begins to roll himself a spindly cigarette.

'Roll us a cig,' says a bloke about my age.

'No you're always bloody cadging and I'm sick of it, I kept you in smokes most of yesterday. So buy your own sodding baccy for a change.'

'Can't you ask your Mam to bring you some in Michael,' says Nancy.

'She aint coming in today.'

'Well go to the canteen and buy yourself some then,' says Bob.

'Ive no dosh till Friday,' says Michael.

'Well look I'll give you one of my cigs but I want it back mind,' Nancy passes Michael a cigarette and turns to me. 'Do you smoke love?' she asks.

I nod my head realising I hadn't had one since yesterday.

'Well you might as well have one as well,' she says offering me the packet, 'but I can't let you have any more, cigs are like bloody gold dust in here.'

Gratefully I take the cigarette and quickly, light it then sit back in the chair inhaling deeply.

You beggar

You despicable bitch.

You've taken that poor woman's cigarette.

As the voices scream out their obscenities I stand up, quickly stub the cigarette out into the over flowing ash tray and scurry away.

Nancy looks on shaking her head. She says something to Bob and I feel their eyes on me. Frantically I start to pace the floor again.

Eventually the voices fade but I carry on walking with my arms wrapped tightly around my stomach.

The nurse pushes the tea trolley into the room and people stand up and form a line besides it and take in turns to pour out their tea.

'Get yourself a cup of tea lass and for god sake stop that aimless wondering up and down, up and down, it's getting on my nerves,' says the old lady I met at breakfast time. She pats the chair next to her, 'come and sit near me.'

Hesitantly I walk towards the seat and sit down taking the pressure from my aching feet.

'Sit back lass and I'll get you a drink. Do you take sugar and milk?'

'Please,' I mutter.

The old lady returns with the tea she hands me the cup of pale brown liquid.

The tea tastes like nectar I drink it fast the hot liquid scalding my throat.

'Feel better now?' asks the old lady with a look of concern.

'Yes, thanks,' I say trying hard to muster a smile.

'That's alright lass we all help each other in here,' she says.

At twelve O'clock prompt everyone stands up and walks towards the dining room.

A smell of stale cabbage insults my nostrils the moment I step into the room.

Once again a queue has formed by the serving hatch so taking a tray I stand in line.

I look down at the food on my plate and my stomach turns at the mound of grey mashed potato, watery cabbage and congealed mincemeat. Pushing the plate away from me I stand up and leave the table.

'You didn't eat a thing, ' says the old woman. 'Wasn't you hungry?'

Sighing I shake my head.

'Can't say I blame you lass,' she mutters

'Lorraine can you join the others in the kitchen,' says a nurse, 'you're on pot duty.

There are two people in the kitchen Nancy stands by an enormous chipped sink busy washing the pots and a man holding a cloth is wiping down surfaces. 'I'm supposed to be here to rest,' sighs Nancy, 'not washing sinks full of dirty dishes.'

'They call it therapy,' mutters the man.

'Some bloody therapy this is, might just as well be at home,' Nancy hands me a tea towel, 'you can dry,' she says.

I take a plate and slowly begin to wipe it with the towel wondering if I'll ever see my home again.

Later that afternoon I watch as an array of people enter the Ward and to my great relief one of them is my Pete.

I sit on his knee by the window and place my head on his shoulder and he gently strokes my hair.
'You'll be alright love, ' he says slowly.
'Where am I? Am, I dead?'
'No you're in hospital but don't worry you're not staying in here for long.'
I move my head off his shoulder. He wipes away a tear from his cheek and looks away.
'What's wrong?' I ask.
'Nothing love,' he says, 'just worry about yourself.'
'Are the bairns safe?'
'The girls are okay so try not to fret.'
'You sure?'
'Of course,' says Pete in a reassuring voice.
Pete holds me close and I stay in his arms until a bell rings.
I look up a nurse is standing by the door.
'Visiting time is over,' she says.
I walk with Pete to the door. He kisses me lightly on the forehead.
'I'll have to go now love,' he says slowly.
He places forty cigarettes in my hand, ruffles my hair and walks out of the door.
That's the last time you'll ever see him, mock the voices.
Sobbing uncontrollably and tightly clutching the packets of cigarettes to me I return to the seat by the window.
'Don't cry love.'.
I look up through a veil of tears and see Nancy standing before me with a box of tissues in her hands. 'What' wrong are you sad because your man has gone home?'
'They told me I'm never going to see him again.' I choke out.
'Who did, the staff?'
'No, no the voices.'
'Do you hear voices love?'

I nod my head.

'Voices in your head?'

'Yes.'

Nancy sighs, 'a lot of people hear voices in here,' she says. 'They play tricks with their heads, best to try to ignore them, .that's what I say. I mean this morning you thought you were dead didn't you'

'I'm not am I.'

'No love you're not you're very much alive.'

I open a packet of cigarettes and offer one to Nancy.

'That's it love sit back and enjoy a smoke and try to ignore those bloody voices they're just a big bag of rubbish. Just think about getting better and going home to your family.'

I want to believe what Nancy has told me, but find I it difficult as the voices seem so real and convincing. And I'm not sure I can put my trust in anyone.

Chapter 5

Despite what the voices say Pete visits every evening. He tells me the kids are doing fine but they can't wait for me to come home. My greatest wish is to be back with my family as I miss them more than anything. And even though Pete insists everything's alright I worry about my babies as I have never been away from them before now.

I sit in the day room watching the old lady do her needlework, her name I've discovered is Rosie. She has a contented look on her face as she nimbly embroiders the edges of a tablecloth. I admire her small intricate stitching. She looks up at me and smiles, her brown eyes crinkle at the corners..
'The doctor says I can go home for a few days next week,' she says.
'I wish I was going home,' I say longingly.
Rosie smiles sympathetically. 'It's a long drawn out process,' she says.
'Do you think they'll let me go home one day?'
'Are you a voluntary patient?'
'I don't know,' I say confused.
'Because if you are you can go home whenever you want, but it's best if you stay here until you're properly better.' Rosie looks down at her sewing and checks the row of stitching 'or sure as eggs are eggs you'll end up coming back,' she says.

I stand up and leave the dayroom.

I knock quietly on the office door.
'Yes Lorraine what do you want,' asks a male nurse.
'Am I a voluntary patient?'
'I believe you are,' says the nurse.
'Well can I go home today?' I say.
Don't trust him!
The nurse sits back in the chair and takes a small pen knife from the top of his pocket.
He's going to kill you.
Startled I cower back.

The nurse looks at me and shakes his head, 'you're far from ready for home yet,' he says as he proceeds to scrape the bowl of his pipe with the penknife. 'You're too paranoid.'

In a daze I walk back to the day room where two nurses are giving out medication from the large cabinet on wheels. A nurse calls out my name and after consulting a file she hands me a cup of water and three tablets. I place them in my mouth and I'm just about to swallow them when the voices in my head screech out their warnings.

Don't do it.

Don't do it.

You are gradually being poisoned.

I turn my head away from the nurses and spit the tablets into a tissue. 'I saw that,' says Bob from the corner of the room, I saw you get rid of your tablets. Rosie looks up from her sewing ,'you should take them,' she tuts 'or you will never get out of here, and you do want to get well don't you?.'

Don't listen to her she knows nothing.

I sit in the day room with the tissue containing the tablets clenched tightly in my hand.

'Take them love,' coaxes Bob, 'then you'll start to feel better.

'But the voices they tell me…..'

'Take no notice of the voices,' says Nancy remember what I told you they're just a big bag of rubbish.'

'Just a part of the illness,' says Bob.

'Think about going home to your bairns.' Says Rosie

Bob gets up from his seat he gives me a can of lemonade and stands watching me whilst I hesitantly put the tablets back in my mouth and swallow them with the lemonade.

'That's it get 'um down your neck love.'

You've done it now.

An icy chill runs down my spine as I stumble out of the room. As I open the door I'm faced with Nurse Margaret.

'Lorraine I've been looking for you,' she says 'the Doctor is on his ward round and he wants to speak with you in his clinic.'

They're six people in the small room they all turn and stare at me as I walk through the door. The doctor sits behind the desk opposite me.

'How do you feel today?' he ask in a deliberately slow voice.

Feeling intimidated by the number of eyes watching me I lower my head.

'I want to go home.'

'From what I hear from the staff I don't think that would be a wise thing at the moment.'

The male nurse I'd seen earlier nods his head in agreement.

'How's your thoughts,' say the doctor, 'tell me what are you thinking of right now.

He's trying to get into my head.' Don't let him in, close your mind don't think about anything make your mind a complete blank.

'Don't you want to speak to me today?'

I stare at the floor..

'And the voices Lorraine, do you still hear them?' the doctor sits back in his chair waiting patiently for my answer.'

Don't tell him anything.

Pay no heed to him.

He despises you.

This is a bad place.

I quickly stand up and scurry out of the room.'

That evening when Pete visits my case is packed ready and waiting.

'But you heard what the doctor said he doesn't think you are ready for home yet,' says the nurse looking at my case. 'Why don't you stay with us a little longer, you can't run away from your problems you know, they're still going to be there when you get home.'

'You can't keep me here,' I say.

Pete nods his head in agreement.

'If you go home against medical advice you will have to sign yourself out and we don't like patients to do that.'

I burst into tears, 'I just want to go home back to my babies,' I cry.

'You won't be much good to your children in the state you're in,' says the nurse.

Pete puts his arm around my shoulders, 'I'm taking my wife home he says.'

After signing the necessary form Pete picks up my case. 'Come on love let's get you out of this place.'

Nancy looks on 'you'll be back lass,' she says shaking her head 'you mark my words you'll be back.'

Chapter 6

The house is quiet Pete is sleeping in his chair and the girls are tucked up safely in their beds. . We picked them up about two hours ago. They had been staying at Pam's.

Their little faces lit up when they saw me. A lump formed in my throat as I held them close, I seemed to have been away from them for so long, so much longer than just one week. I look around my living room it seems so tiny compared to the hospital ward. I hug myself as it feels so good to be back here in my own home.

Pete is going to take a week off work. He says we are going to spend some time together. This pleases me because I feel a rest will do him good. With three little ones money's a bit tight so Pete usually works all the hours God sends.

I look across at Pete he stirs in his sleep and then his eyes flick open as though aware of my presence, his eyes meet mine.

'You okay love?' he says do you fancy a cup of tea?'

'It's alright Pete I'll make it,' I stand up and walk into the kitchen.

Pete follows me, 'you may as well have your tablets now,' he says as he opens the small brown bottle I had been given when I left the hospital.

Pete then hands me my tablets and a glass of water.

Remembering what Nancy had told me I quickly swallow them back with the water.

Smiling to myself I fill the kettle put it on the stove and light a cigarette,

She thinks she's the queen of the castle.
She's an idiot.
A simple bitch.

Trying hard to ignore the voices I get the cups from the cupboard.

My hand shakes as I reach for the glass sugar bowl. I drop it; there is spilt sugar and glass all over the kitchen floor.

Clumsy cow isn't she.

I burst into tears.

Pete puts his arm around me 'oh don't worry about that love,' he says when he sees the mess on the floor. 'Go and put your feet up, 'I'll make the tea.'

I sit down on the sofa with tears streaming down my face as the voices rattle on inside my head.

Clumsy cow.

Useless fool.

She isn't fit for mankind.

Pete returns from the kitchen carrying the mugs of tea.

'Oh it's only a bit of sugar love don't cry,' he says.

'I'm frightened.'

Pete sits by my side on the sofa, he holds me close

Don't be scared love, I'm here I'll look after you.

'Am I alright?'

'You're going to be fine love you're with me now.'

Pete takes me in his arms and I stay for some time there until the voices gradually fade away and I start to feel a little safer.

'That's it love, try and relax, I think you've been overdoing things a bit what with the house and the kids and everything. '

I sigh wishing things were that simple.

Later that night lying in my own bed listening to the rain pattering on the windows and Pete's rhythmical snores I feel a sense of peace drift over me as I'm lulled into slumber.

It doesn't feel like I'd been sleeping long when I'm woken up by the shrilling of the alarm clock. I sit up and stretch feeling refreshed for the first time in weeks.

The door opens and Cheryl trundles through it sleepy eyed and hazy. She climbs in the bed between me and Pete and snuggles into me.

'I'm glad your home Mammy,' she says 'I missed you so much.'

'I have you me little love,' I kiss her soft head.'

'Come on you two it's time we were getting up,' smiles Pete.

'Mam?' asks Lucy over breakfast 'can I have the day off school today I know you've been poorly and I want to stay at home and look after you.'

'You've got to go to school love ,'says Pete. 'But don't worry about your Mam I'll look after her.'

Sammy looks up at me her big blue eye search my face. 'You'll still be here when we get home won't you Mam?' she says.

'Of course she will love,' says Pete, 'she's home now.'

I give Sammy a reassuring look and she smiles with relief.

Lucy is the first to leave the house she's eleven now and has recently started to attend the senior school.

I stand on the step and wave her of
Presently Pete and I take our two younger children to the local primary.

'You look so much better today,' says Pete when we return, 'not so tired, did you have a good night's sleep?'
'Best night I've had in ages.'
'It's nice when it's just me and you isn't it I mean the kids are great but we never have any time together it's all bed and bloody work as a rule, ' says Pete

******

Later on that morning I call my Mam and I apologise to her.
'It's okay love,' she says. 'I know you're not well I'm more worried about you than anything and I don't think you should have signed yourself out of the hospital times young yet.'

******

Over the next few days try as I might I can't dismiss the strange thought that enters my mind. I feel as though I've been punished for something. However the voices are not so prominent and I feel a little safer while Pete's around. But all too soon the week is over and it's time for Pete to go back to work.

Chapter 7

I walk around the house in a daze Pete went to work about an hour ago and it's nearly time to get the kids up for school. I don't really want them to go I worry about their safety.   The sink is full of unwashed pots and there's a pile of clothes on the sofa waiting to be ironed. There's so much to do and I don't know where to start so I sit in the chair and smoke two cigarettes. Eventually I can hear Lucy in the bathroom and then I hear the sounds of Sammy and Cheryl coming down the stairs.

'Morning Mam,' says Sammy as she enters the room Cheryl follows close behind her.

I go through the motions of getting the breakfast ready but Cheryl doesn't want any and Sammy spills her juice all over the carpet.

Lucy finally arrives from the bathroom looking so much older than her eleven years. She has her hair done different to how she normally does and is wearing a trace of lipstick. A lump form in my throat.

Sammy takes one look at Lucy, you look stupid,' she says

Lucy and Sammy then get into an argument which seems to last for ages.

It takes me some time to sort the argument out but eventually peace is restored.

Lucy then leaves for school in a huff.

'Mammy we're going to be late for school,' says Sammy looking at the clock on the mantel piece. 'The little handle's nearly on the nine and that's when the whistle goes.'

Sammy and Cheryl are still in their pyjamas.

I look at the pile of clothes on the sofa and realise that I haven't ironed the school clothes.

Bad mother, bad mother. Chant the voices.

I quickly assemble the ironing board trapping my finger in the process, plug in the iron and quickly run it over the clothes but I can't get the pleats in Sammy's skirt to look right.

Useless Bitch.

Bad Mother.

'Mammy why are you crying?' says Cheryl.

'Oh it's nothing love come on let's get you ready for school.

I quickly help the girls to dress in the newly ironed clothes. After we have hastily put on our shoes and coats we leave the house.

'Whistle will have gone ages ago,' says Sammy.'
'We're going to be very late,' says Cheryl.
My legs feel like jelly as we walk down the street, we pass a man who seems to look right through me. My heart pounds. The voices laugh and cackle inside my head.
A group of woman stand by the telephone box talking they glare at me in contempt, I shudder.
Everyone hates you.
You're bad.
Despicable bitch.
We reach the side of the road, a dog barks it's anger at me.
'Hey Lorraine what's wrong you don't look well,' says the lollipop lady.
'Mammy's been poorly,' says Cheryl.
Ignoring the lollipop lady I see the kids across the road.
The school is in sight now.
'We can go the rest of the way ourselves now mam,' says Sammy.
The kids then run on in front.
Bad mother.
Evil.
Sweat pours down my face and in a panic I turn and run..
I reach the road and don't stop running, brakes screech.
'Hey what's the rush?' says the lollipop lady, 'that car almost hit you.'
I pass the group of women standing by the telephone box they look my way..
'What the hell's up with her?'
'Looks like she's got the fear of God in her.'
They titter and carry on talking.
I reach my house and quickly let myself in and lock the door behind me. I then retreat to my chair in the living room and franticly light another cigarette after about an hour the ashtray is full.
The doorbell rings I let it ring for some time before I pluck up the courage to answer it.
Pam stands on my step.
'What's the door doing locked? She says as she steps into the house.
'I'm frightened.'.
'Well you've got no reason to be frightened so why don't you try and pull yourself together for the kids sake, it's only your nerves.'
She sits on the edge of the sofa.

'I've just come to see how you're getting on,' she looks around the room with distaste in her eyes.

'Why don't you get on with your housework,' she says 'there's nothing better for your nerves than housework.

'I'm a bad mother.'

'Well you're not much good to them right now,' says Pam, 'like I say pull yourself together you're a married women turned thirty not a child.'

'Am I wicked.'

Pam's eyes roll towards the ceiling.

'Yes,' she says with a smirk, 'you are, fancy getting the police out on your own Mother.'   Pam stands up, 'well I'll be going now so get on with your work and don't sit drinking cups of tea all day with that Jane. I might come back later and see how you're getting on.'

Feeling like a naughty school child I sit in my chair and once again resort to my cigarettes.

You useless lazy bastard.

You're going to die.

Hell is waiting for you.

My whole body trembles as I rock back and forth in my chair.

You good for nothing bitch.

I nip my wrist until the skin goes bright red and clenching my fist tightly I begin to punch myself in the head.   And the voices erupt into harsh laughter.

We've got her now.

We've got her now.

She's ours now

In an effort to drown out the voices, I flick on the radio and turn up the volume.

I listen to the record been played. '*I can see Clearly now the rain has gone.*'

The song comes to an end.

I can see clearly now Lorraine has gone, taunt the voices, before breaking off into more hideous laughter.

I run up the stairs and enter my bedroom I get in to the bed lie and lay there with the blankets pulled tightly over my head. After some time the laughter dies down until it gradually stops.

I don't know how long I have been lying here. I may have fallen asleep the radio is still playing down the stairs. I get out of bed shame washes over me as I peel the wet sheets off the soaked mattress.

Having changed out of my damp clothes I return back down the stairs and turn off the radio.

I then leave the house and scurry with my head down to my mams house. I open the door, my Mam is sitting on the sofa. She looks up and smiles warmly at me.

'I'm having a bad day Mam,' I say and I just can't cope.' I burst into tears.

'Oh come and sit down love,' my Mam patts the side of the sofa near where she is sitting.

I sit by her side and rest my head on her shoulder.

'I'm going to take you to the doctors. Perhaps he can give you some stronger tablets or you might feel a little better just to have a chat with him.'

The doctor's waiting room is almost empty and almost as soon as we sit down my name is called out by the receptionist.

'Do you want me to come in the surgery with you?' asks my Mam.

'No I'll be okay.'

'Well don't forget to tell the doctor everything that's bothering you.'

'Take a seat,' says Doctor Harris, pointing to the chair opposite him.

I sit down facing him..

'How can I help you?

I lower my head, the doctor waits for me to answer but I say nothing.

'Lorraine would you like to tell me why you've come here today,' says the doctor breaking the silence.

I think it's my nerves,' I say slowly.

'I see,' says Doctor Harris 'how have you coped since you left the hospital?.'

I look up to see the doctors eyes are warm and full of sympathy.

I try to hold back my tears but can do nothing to stop them from falling down my face.

The doctor hands me a box of tissues, 'you appear to be very anxious are you still hearing voices?'

'Yes I mutter,' in a small voice.

'When did you last hear them?'

'This morning.'

'Would you like to tell me what they say to you?'

I shake my head.

'Have you been taking your tablet regularly?'

'Yes,' I mutter.

'Then they may start working soon, they usually take about three weeks before they get in your system. But if they don't make you feel any better we can change them for you.' The doctor looks up at me and smiles kindly, 'we'll get you a community psychiatric nurse . I'll arrange for her to visit you, but you can come back and see me anytime you feel you need to.'

My mam's waiting for me in the waiting room, 'do you feel a bit better now you've had a little chat? she asks her voice full of concern.

'Yeah I'm okay Mam,' I say not wanting to worry her anymore.

My mam looks relieved. We walk down the road, and stop outside her house,

'There's no need for you to go back home to sit brooding on your own,' she says., 'you may as well come back and sit with me for a few hours..'

The first thing I see when we enter the home where I spent part of my childhood are packing boxes. My dad is busy wrapping ornaments in newspaper. . Much to my Mam's joy they had recently sold the house and were due to be moving in a couple of weeks.

I know I will miss her desperately, but then I tell myself, she will only be a bus ride away and I feel pleased for her because I know how much she wants to retire to the country.

I follow my Mam as she carries the tea tray into the living room, we both sit down by the glowing fire.

'Try not to worry too much,' says my Mam in between sip of her tea 'you were poorly like this before and had to go to that hospital but you got well and you will again.'

I think back over the years to when I was fifteen. I recall the experience that I suffered through then. An experience which up until now had been buried deep.

One that I'd pushed to the back of my mind and had not allowed it to rear itself. It was a terrible time which was also filled with fear and uncertainty where the voices raged and laughed inside my head. Although I'd eventually returned to what I considered reality. Now that the voices and horrible distressing thoughts are back my confusion as to what reality really is has grown and both are beginning to merge.

Chapter 8

Over the next two days my confusion deepens until I can't concentrate for long on anything.

My Psychiatric nurse visited me and although she tried her best she couldn't ease my troubled mind and dispel the disturbing thoughts I have.

She gave me a relaxation tape to play, I played it a couple of times but it did nothing to silence the voices and stop my fears.

It's got now so that I just can't cope with everyday life.

Pam had to pick my babies up this morning and take them to school as I've become too afraid to leave the house.

And as the housework piles up around me my feelings of worthlessness intensify.

The kitchen has taken on a smell of damp washing and neglect I look at the mound of dirty clothes on the floor and decide to try and to do something about it.

Using what energy I can muster I pull the twin-tub out from beneath the sink, attach the rubber pipe to the tap and proceed to fill up the drum with hot water.

I then add some of the dirty washing it is badly stained some of it having black mould on it after being left damp on the kitchen floor for too long.

Sighing I add the powder and turn on the machine. I watch as the agitator swishes the washing around the drum and I begin to feel a little comforted.

Two hours later the washing is finished. I feel pleased with my accomplishment.

Plucking up my courage I open the back door and taking my peg bag I drag the wash basket containing the newly washed clothes towards the washing line in my garden.

The sweat pours down my back as I hang the washing on the line. My mouth feels dry and I feel sick so I hang the clothes out as quickly as I can. Two sheets are stained with tiny black flecks left from the mould but I leave them hanging there on the line and retreat back indoors..

I sit by the window looking at the stained sheets as they flap in the wind.

You filthy bitch.
You're a failure.
You will be reported to the authorities for hanging dirty washing on the line.
You're going to get it.
You've done it now.
Disgusting slattern.

As the voices spit out their threats I stare out of the window and watch as the rain begins to fall from the grey sky.

The long hours pass I stay in the chair until the voices diminish and all I can hear is the rain as it splashes on the window. Using all the courage I can muster I stand up go to the back door, open it and step into the garden.
My washing hangs heavy and saturated on the line. Before I have managed to retrieve it the washing line suddenly snaps. With tears falling down my face I pick up the sodden clothes from the muddy garden and carry them into the house where I drop them back in a heap on to the kitchen floor.

******

'Mammy there was no one to meet us at the school gate and we had to come home all by ourselves.' Says Cheryl as she walks in the door.
'Don't worry Mam we came straight home and we didn't talk to strangers,' says Sammy.
My face burns with shame when I realise that I'd forgotten to make arrangements for them to be picked up, *the voices are right I am a bad mother.*

Chapter 9

'I wish I could get to the bottom of what's bothering you love,' says Pete.

I sit on the sofa and fix my gaze on a focus point in the corner of the room.

'Can't you just tell me what's on your mind?'

Don't trust that Man.

He despises you.

I quickly move away from the sofa and sit on a hard backed chair.

Pete sighs deeply, 'I wish you would snap out of it,' He stares at the wall and we sit in silence.

The clock ticks away on the mantelpiece and I count the seconds.

When I reach one thousand I stand up and walk out of the room.

I lie in bed and will myself to sleep wanting desperately to escape from the turmoil and fear.

Presently I hear Pete coming up the stairs. He enters our bedroom and climbs into bed beside me. He gently places his arm around me but I turn around and move to the edge of our bed and begin counting again.

******

I've been lying here for hours praying for sleep to release me from my guilt and the disturbing thoughts that cloud my mind. I know I'm going to be punished for my inadequacies, my failure to protect my babies, and that very soon the authorities will catch up with me and I will be at their mercy.

Dawn is almost breaking and I lie there listening as the birds wake up.

'Bad Bad,' croaks the angry crow.

'You must be joking you must be joking,' twitter the sparrows.

I sit up quickly, the early morning sun filters through the grubby net curtains.

I shudder another day has begun.

Pete grunts in his sleep as I climb out of bed. On tiptoe I leave the bedroom and steal down the stairs.

******

I stand in the kitchen with the bread knife held close to my wrist; I stare at my veins and lower the knife down until it's almost touching my skin. I then think of my family sleeping peacefully upstairs in their beds and of them waking up to find me lifeless and covered in blood. Ashamed of myself and afraid of my own actions I quickly place the knife back in the drawer and scurry out of the kitchen..
Coward.
I stand by the living room door looking at the sideboard.
My babies smile at me from framed photographs. Memories of happier days when things were so simple. Times I had taken for granted flash through my mind.

Enveloped in sadness I sit in my chair where I silently pray for those times to return.

Consumed with guilt I think about what I'd almost done. A lump forms in my throat and my mouth feels dry and parched. I need to quench my thirst but I'm too afraid to go back into the kitchen to get a drink of water.
My eyes then rest on my ornaments, little knick knacks I collected over the years, treasures Pete and the girls had bought me for birthdays and Christmas.
You're not worthy of anything.
You don't deserve happiness.
The room spins round, my head throbs and the voices screech, and the lump in my throat is getting bigger. I walk up to the sideboard it's inches thick in dust and grime.
Slattern.
Slovenly bitch.
You're not worthy.
You're not worthy.
Sobs catch in my throat as I pick up an armful of ornaments and throw them at the wall. With tears streaming down my face I carry on until every single ornament is smashed.

'What the bloody hell's going on,' says Pete as he enters the room. He then stops dead in his tracks and takes one look at the smashed up ornaments, 'Oh Lorraine,' he says what the hell have you done that for?'
I sit in the middle of the floor rocking myself backwards and forwards.

'I'm not worthy,' I mutter, 'I'm bad the voices are right.

'You're not making sense love,' Pete walks across the room and tries to take my in his arms.
'Go away!' I scream pushing him away 'I'm not worthy.'
The morning passes. Pete makes me a cup of tea but I ignore him and leave the tea to go cold.
'You better try and pull yourself together love,' says Pete 'the kids will be getting up soon and you don't want them to see you in this state.'
'I'm not worthy,' I mutter.
Pete sighs, 'why don't you go back to bed, 'you might feel better after a rest, don't worry about the kids I'll take the day off work.'
Obeying him I stand up and walk out of the room.

Feeling utterly worthless I lie in bed listening as Pete gets the girls ready for school.'
'Where's me Mammy,' I hear Cheryl say.
'You're Mammy's in bed poorly.'
'Can I go and kiss her better Daddy.'
'No, let her rest love.'
'Will she still be here when we get back home?'
'I'm not sure Sammy.'
'Will she ever get better?'
'Yeah course she will Lucy love, I'll get the doctor out today he may be able to give her some better tablets.'
'Will she have to go back to hospital?'
'Yes love,' says Pete, 'she might.'
The bleating of a car horn fills my ears..
'Come on kids,' I hear Pete say that'll be Pam.'
I walk to the windows and look out watching as my girls clamber Pam's car. I never even kissed them goodbye. I may not see them again, the authorities are coming to get me.
I watch until the car containing my babies is out of view.

Bad Mother, hiss the voices.
Too lazy to take her kids to school.
Useless.
She's not fit for man nor beast.
Feeling numb and empty inside I lie back on the bed.

Presently I hear Pete's footsteps on the stairs, the bedroom door opens slowly and he enters the bedroom.

'I think it will be for the best love,' he says if we can get a doctor to see you,' I just didn't realise how sick you are. Perhaps you shouldn't have signed yourself out of the hospital and maybe it will be for the best if you go back in again until they've got your head sorted out.'

'You can do what you like with me,' I mutter, 'I'm just no good.'

******

Doctor Harris sits on the sofa alongside him sits a man who has introduced himself as Doctor Spencer consultant psychiatrist.

'How are you feeling today Lorraine? he asked, 'I understand from what your husband's just told me that you're not too well.

Don't look at that man.

He's reading your mind.

I avert my eyes and look down at the carpet.

'Can you tell me why you smashed your ornaments up?' asks Doctor Spencer.

I say nothing and try to keep my mind a complete blank.

'Can you tell me what you're thinking of right now?'

I close my eyes tightly listening to the voices having a conversation about me.

She's older than time

She's been here before.

She's the chosen one.

She's wicked.

'Lorraine can you hear me?' says Doctor Spencer.

I look up and nod my head.

'Can you tell me how old you are.'

'I'm older than time,' I say.

'What makes you say that?' Asks Doctor Harris.

'The voices,' I mutter half to myself.

Doctor Spencer writes something down in a file, 'do you hear voices Lorraine?' he asks.

Slowly I nod my head.

Doctor Harris smiles sympathetically but I'm not fooled.

'I think,' says Doctor Spencer looking up that you should be readmitted to hospital I'll make the necessary arrangements.

I think it will be for the best Doctor,' says Pete sighing.

I shrug my shoulders knowing it will be futile to argue.

The ambulance arrives about half an hour later and like a little lamb to the slaughter I'm led up the path towards its open doors.

Chapter 10

A mixture of fear and sadness grips my stomach as I pace up and down the hospital ward.

'Come and sit with us love,' says Nancy. She walks up to me, takes my hand and leads me to a chair. The group of people look on, some of them smile whilst others seem to look through me with glassy eyes and vacant expressions.

Nancy sighs, 'I told you that you'd be back here, didn't I love?' she says 'are you going to stop in now until you're properly better?'

'What's my babies going to do' I say bursting into tears they'll never see me again I'm a bad mother. The authorities are going to punish me.'

Nancy shakes her head, 'are you still listening to those voices,' she says.

'Have they put your children in care love,' says a women of about my age,

'they did that to mine.'

'I'm a failure.'

'Of course you're not,' says Nancy, 'you're not in here to be punished you're in here to get well just like the rest of us. I know it's not the best place in the world but you're in the right place right now. So if you just take your tablets and stop listening to those voices you should soon start feeling better, and then you'll be able to go back home to your little family.'

Don't trust that woman she knows nothing.

I stand up and walk away.

With tears stinging my cheeks I begin to pace the floor again.

Let me die to take to away the pain let me go to release me from the fear that grips my soul in a cold fist. For I'm the chosen one and they will come in the middle of the night when all is quiet and I will be tortured slowly........

The voices screech mockingly as they read my deepest thoughts.

'What's my babies going to do now,' I cry. 'I'm never going to see them again.'

'Stop being so bloody pathetic and either sit your arse down or piss off,' says a man sitting by the door. 'I can't be doing with listening to whining depressed bloody women.'

'Leave the lass alone,' says a women sitting nearby, 'you was in hell of a state too when you was first admitted.'

'Well I'll be glad to be getting out of this nuthouse in a couple of days,' says the man.

'Did you hear that,' smiles the woman, 'he's going home soon and you will as soon as you're better, so you will see your kids again.'

Pay no heed to the woman.

She lies; you will be in here forever and a day.

My heart beating rapidly I make my way to the door.

'Where are you going?' says a nurse.

'I want to go home,' I say.

'You've only just come Lorraine, come with me and we'll go and have a little chat.'

I follow the nurse down a short corridor and into a room.

'Sit down and try to relax,'

With bated breath I sit on the edge of the chair.

The authorities have sent her to spy on you.

Be careful be careful.

Keep your mind blank don't look at her she's reading your thoughts don't let her into your head................

'You seem very anxious,' says the nurse, 'how long have you been feeling like this?'

I close my eyes tightly trying desperately to clear my mind, *12345678910,* I fill my head with numbers and the clock on the wall ticks away the seconds.

'Don't you want to talk with me Lorraine?'

 Ignore her don't look into her eyes, she' out to get you.

The nurse smiles but I can see through her and I know it's all pretence a sly trick to deceive me into believing I'm safe.

''You've been here before haven't you?' she says.

I swallow back the saliva in my mouth for those were the exact words the voices used.

I look up and nod my head quickly, 'yes I'm older than time,' I say.almost to myself.

The nurse smiles again as though she hasn't heard me, 'the doctor will be on the ward soon,' she says, 'he may give you something to settle you.'

We sit in the quite room for some time The nurse tries her best to assure me and make conversation but I stare at the floor biting the sides of my mouth.

******

'She seems very anxious and yet unresponsive Doctor,' says the nurse.

The Doctor looks at me over the top of his horn rimmed spectacles, ' Lorraine he says slowly is there anything at all on your mind?'

I ignore him.

'Are you still hearing voices? '

There is an awkward pause whilst the doctor waits for my answer.

Don't say anything.

Don't you want to speak to me Lorraine.?'

Being careful not to meet his eyes I shake my head and walk out of the room..

'We'll try again tomorrow,' I hear the doctor say before I close the door.

I walk back down the corridor and return back to the ward where I sit alone at the far end of the room, away from the vacant stares and the endless chit –chat.

Later that evening I watch as the medicine trolley is pushed on to the ward. Eventually my name is called so with trembling legs I walk towards the nurse who is giving out the tablets.

She looks up at me and smiles.

'I think what you need most of all is a good night's sleep,' she says, 'the doctor has written down something that will help to relax you, but in order for them to work you must go straight to bed.'

I take the tablets quickly and another nurse takes me upstairs to the dormitory and shows me where my bed is.

'Get change into your night clothes, and try and get some sleep she says, before she leaves the room.

I sit on the edge of the bed.

Don't lay down don't close your eyes stay awake for tonight they may come and get you........

My heart pounding I blink away the sleep that pricks my eyelids I can hear someone coming up the stairs. I feel the hair stand up at the back of my neck as the dormitory door is opened.

I watch as people enter the dormitory.

'Are you still awake?' asks Nancy as she climbs in the bed opposite me I thought you'd be in the land of nod by now.'

Nancy looks across at me, 'bloody hell she says what on earths wrong you look terrified.'

Feeling too choked up to speak I stay where I am on the edge of my bed.

'Nurse nurse!' Shouts Nancy, Lorraine isn't well in fact she looks to me like she's going to pass out.'

The nurse walks up to me, 'get into bed and lie down.' She says gently.

'She looks scared out of her wits,' says Nancy.

Slowly I get into bed.

'Lie down,' says the nurse, 'there's no need to be afraid.'

Exhausted I lie back on the pillows, the nurse holds my hand 'I'm going to stay here by your side until you're asleep,' she says. 'So close your eyes and think about nice things.'

Her hand feels soft and warm and her voice is reassuring.

'Aren't they coming tonight,' I ask, 'aren't they coming to get me.'

'You're quite safe here Lorraine,' soothes the nurse, I think you've just been imagining things.'

'Am I to be punished?'

'No you're just in here to get well, no one's going to hurt you. Hush now close your eyes, that's it relax.'

I breathe a sigh of relief.

My baby is lying in her crib, her first smile lights up her face. I pick her up and nestle her to my breast. Her big blue eyes gaze adoringly into mine as she feeds. I look back at her in wonder and I can't believe she's mine..............

'Morning!' shouts a chirpy voice.

I sit up and look around me, tears stream down my cheeks as I realise that I'd just been dreaming. My arms feel empty and my heart aches I feel as though something inside of me has died, a precious time which I know will never come back.

'Well that's a right way to greet the morning isn't it,' said a nurse looking at my face.

'Come on let's have you up you'll feel better when you've had a little wash.'

I take my change of clothes and follow the shuffling women to the bathroom.

I stand at the sink and splash the warm water on my face. A woman stands at the sink beside me brushing her teeth.

The bathroom door opens and two nurses enter carrying an old lady. One nurse holds her by her wrists and the other one has hold of her thin ankles. The old lady has her eyes tightly closed as though still in a deep sleep.

The woman by my side finishes brushing her teeth and looks on, 'that's Madge,' she says, 'she won't get up in a morning. That's why they have to carry her from her bed and to the bathroom still half asleep.'

The woman looks towards the old lady, 'you'd sleep all day if they let you wouldn't you Madge,' she laughs.

Longing for some privacy I take off my nightdress, wash the rest of my body, put on my clothes I leave the bathroom as quickly as I can. I go back to the dormitory realising I'd left my handbag containing my cigarettes in my locker..

Nancy is making her bed, 'We all have to make our own bed in here,' she says looking at my rumpled up covers. 'Would you like me to show you how to do it properly I've been here long enough to know how they like it done.'

Without waiting for an answer Nancy strips my bed and in no time she efficiently demonstrates how to make neat hospital corners. 'I smile my thanks take my handbag and leave the dormitory

The day room is full of people. An old man sitting smoking a pipe reminds me of my grandad, I sit by his side and take my packet of number six king size from my handbag. My head throbs and my mouth feels dry like sandpaper. Despite this I light the cigarette.

'Have you got a cig I can borrow?' says a girl, 'I'm bloody gasping.'

'Bugger off Angie' says the old man, 'you're always bloody cadging cigs you'd pinch me pipe if I let you.'

Angie hovers around me until I hand her a cig when without a word of thanks she takes it and walks away.

'You'll never have her off your back now,' says the man, 'she's the biggest cadger in here.' The old man looks at me and I can see my face reflected in his watery blue eyes. 'There's something familiar about you,' he says. 'Have you been here before?'

His words echo around my head *have you been here before have you been here before.*

Trembling I inhale deeply on my cigarette.

Chapter 11

I watch as people begin the enter the ward and to my joy one of them is my Pete

'Do you feel any better love?' he asks as he sits by my side. I get up from my chair and sit on his knee he holds me gently in his arms and plants a soft kiss on my forehead.

'The nurse tells me you had a good night's sleep last night,' he says.

'Are my babies' alright?'

'Yes there're fine Pam is looking after them but they can't wait for you to get well again and come home.'

I swallow back the lump in my throat, 'will I be able to come home one day?' I ask.

'Of course you will love, you don't think I'd let them keep you in this place do you.'

'But the voices they say...................'

'The voices aren't real love so take no notice of them.'

'Am I sick?'

'Yes you are and you must start accepting that.'

'But the voices they tell me............'

Pete sighs, 'there not real, try to ignore them, concentrate on getting well and coming home again.'

I point to the old man in the corner, 'he knows,' I say, 'he knows I've been here before because I'm old much older than he is.'

'Pete holds me tighter, 'don't be silly Lorraine you're only just turned thirty that man must be pushing eighty.'

'I'm older than time,' I say.

'You're just confused love I suppose it's a part of the illness he mutters half to himself.

I stay in Pete's arms, he strokes my hair and we sit in silence until the bell goes signalling the end of visiting time.

'Now I don't want you to get upset or worry about anything,' Pete stands up. If you need to talk to someone and I'm not in you can talk to your Mam or your brother Grahame.' He hands me a piece of paper which contain their telephone numbers and a small bag containing twenty pence coins.

After kissing me quickly on the cheek Pete leaves the ward.

I look down at the piece of paper I have in my hand.
Rip it up. Hiss the voices.

No one wants to talk to you.
Biting the sides of my mouth I ignore the voices and put the piece of paper in my back pocket.
Your wicked.
Evil.
A wicked bitch of a witch.

My head throbs as I run down the corridor towards the payphone. Before I lose my courage I pick up the receiver drop in a coin and quickly dial my brother's telephone number. I hear crackling in my ear and I'm just about to put down the receiver when my brother answers.
'Who's speaking?' says Grahame.'
'It's me Lorraine.'
'Hiya Lorraine how you doing I hear you're not very well.'
'Am I wicked?'
I hear Grahame cough. 'No don't be daft,' he says.
'The voices tell me I am they say I'm evil.'
'What voices?'
'In my head, I'm frightened.'
'But they're' in your head, the voices can't hurt you and what they're saying to you isn't true because you haven't got a wicked bone in your body.'
'Do you hate me?'
'No we all love you Lorraine and want you to get well. There's just something wrong with your brain right now.'
'But the voices_____ I'm scared. Grahame.'
'Tell the voices to Fuck off, like I say they can't hurt you so fight the bastards and tell them to fuck off.'
'Am I bad?'
'No Lorraine, 'you're a good lass and I know how brave you are so tell them voices to fuck off. Anyway Lorraine I'm coming to see you in a couple of days so just try to hang on in there and don't forget what I said..'
'I don't know_____ I'
'You   must   fight   'em'   fight   'em'   tooth   and   nail   don't_____'
'Grahame, Grahame, the line cackles and goes dead so I quickly place the receiver back down on its cradle and return to the ward.

The evening passes and before I know it it's bedtime again.

Thankful that the day has come to an end I lie in bed but sleep doesn't come and free me from the thoughts that are running round and round in my mind; terrible thoughts which are impossible to dismiss. Despite what Pete had said to me during visiting time I wonder if I will ever get out of this strange place, and most of all if I will ever see my babies again. I believe that the voices are real and apart from the tricks they play I feel that most of what they say to me is true. Perhaps I was wicked in another life and today I have to pay for my past sins. I think of my inadequateness and my failures as a woman and a mother and I pray that one day I get the chance to go home and try again.

Unable to lie there any longer I leave my bed take my cigarettes and go into the day room. A nurse is sitting in the corner, she looks at me and sighs.

'What are you doing up?' she says, 'it's two thirty in the morning you should be sleeping.'

'I can't sleep,' I mutter, taking a cigarette from my packet I hastily light it.

'Well I can't give you a sleeping tablet tonight,' she says, 'the doctor only wrote you down for one last night he says tonight you must try and have some natural sleep.'

The nurse sits back in her chair she also lights a cigarette, 'don't tell anyone you've seen me smoking in here,' she says 'or you'll get me hung.'

I look at the nurse, she seems more human somehow with a cigarette dangling between her lips.

'Is there anything bothering you that's stopping you from sleeping, you look very sad.'

'I'll never see them again,' I mutter with a sob catching in my throat.

'Who's that?' says the nurse.

'My babies.'

'Why's that then?

I'll never get out of here.'

'Of course you will as soon as you're well.'

Don't trust her.

She's out to get you.

The nurse looks at me closely 'and we will get you better so try not to get upset'

She's lying.

You'll never go home again.

'Fuck off.' I mumble under my breath.

The nurse crunches her cigarette out in the over flowing ash tray, 'you've got to learn to trust people,' she says before she leaves the room.

You're nothing but a fool.

'Fuck off,' I say a little louder the voices then erupt into mocking laughter.

Overcome with frustration I pick up the ashtray and hurl it towards the wall, tab ends spew on to the grey carpet as the ashtray smashes into several pieces.

The nurse comes back into the room, sighing and shaking her head she proceeds to pick up the broken glass. 'You can just get yourself back to bed.' She says.

I've been lying in bed for what seems like hours before I hear the dormitory come to life. Nancy is the first to wake up and together we go into the bathroom having washed and dressed we go down the stairs and into the smoke room.

'Bloody hell you've got big bags under your eyes,' says Nancy. ' Have you had a bad night love?'

I nod my head.

'Never mind you'll settle in soon, perhaps you need some fresh air. If you want we could go for a little walk on the grounds today, or maybe go to the canteen for a cuppa. Would you like that?'

'Will they let me out,' I ask hesitantly.

'Of course they will, you're not a bloody prisoner.'

****

Nancy puts her arm in mine, 'we'll go and have a cuppa first,' she says, 'and then we'll go for nice walk in the grounds. It'll do you world of good, much better than been stuck on the ward all day long.'

The canteen is inside the main building and a group of people stand outside. A tall man walks up to me he has his grey hair slicked back into quiff and is wearing strange coat.

'That's Tom,' mutters Nancy, 'he a teddy- boy.'

'Hiya Nancy,' says Tom, 'whose your friend?'

'Her name's Lorraine,' says Nancy.

Tom smiles at me and looks me up and down I begin to feel uneasy, 'will you be my woman?'

Shaking my head I step back.'

'She's spoken for,' laughs Nancy.
We enter the main building and pass reception, to the left is the door to the canteen.
'You don't want to be scared of Tom,' says Nancy, he's only being friendly, been in here for years he has.'
When we enter the canteen a strange sickly smell hits my nostrils. Cigarette smoke hangs in smoggy tendrils above tables that are littered with dirty cups. We get a cup of watery grey tea from the vending machine in the corner. And sit down at oneof the tables someone has spat in the middle of it I look at the white frothy pool of phlegm and I shudder.
A middle aged woman also dressed in the fashions of the fifties joins us at the table.
She picks up a tab-end from the overflowing ashtray and attempts' to light it. I offer her one of my cigarettes her eyes lighting up she takes it from my packet.
'Don't start that,' says Nancy, 'or you'll have none left.'
Almost on cue our table is surrounded by people, 'gis a cigg, giss a gig, they all say in unison.
I give each one of them a number six. They light it quickly and look on as though I'd just given them the world.
I look down at my packet I only have two cigs left.
'What did I tell you,' sighs Nancy, 'now you'll l have to make them last right until your husband brings you some more.'
I sigh wondering how I'm going to manage.
'Never mind,' says Nancy looking at my face, 'I'll lend you some of mine.'
We sit in the canteen for some time and drink our tea.. An old record plays in the background and Tom taps his feet in time to the music. I look out of the window the morning sun has now been covered by the grey clouds.
'I think,' says Nancy following my gaze, 'that we should go for our walk now before it pisses down.,
I nod my head in agreement and together Nancy and I leave the canteen.
'We'll go and see the horses, 'there's some in at field the end of the drive, they don't belong to the hospital but I often go and see them.'
We walk along the long drive towards the back entrance.

We have walked about half way down when we come to a large building it has a veranda with tables chairs. I stop outside and look towards it. My mind flashes back to when I was fifteen.

'That's Sledmere ward,' says Nancy.

'I know,' I reply slowly, 'I was in here once.'

'When was that?'

'Oh a real long time ago when I was a young girl.'

'So you've been ill before?'

'I think so, but I'd rather not talk about it.'

I look towards Sledmere Ward,   suppressed memories come to the foe and I want to be sick.

Nancy takes my arm, 'come on,' she says gently, 'let's go and see those horses.'

Sighing I walk away from Sledmere ward.

We watch from the gate, the horses run around the field. One of them has rolled on to its back and is   kicking its legs into the air. I sigh to myself and envy their freedom.

We stay by the gate until the first drops of rain fall from the sky.

'Let's get back to the ward now,' says Nancy, 'otherwise we'll get soaked.'

With my head down I walk back up the long drive increasing my pace when I pass Sledmere ward with all its memories.

The rain falls down faster and as I scurry along the laughter starts up inside my head.

'Are you alright?' says Nancy in between breaths as she tries to keep up with me.

You'll never be right, cackle the voices.

You're bad.

'Fuck of,' I say.

'What was that?' says Nancy, 'what did you just say?'

Wicked bitch

Fuck off,' I say louder.

'Don't tell me to fuck off,' says Nancy, 'there's no bloody need for that.'

I run on leaving Nancy behind. I reach the side entrance of Garton ward I run across the field opposite it. In the distance I can see a small church, I run across anther field which leads to a dirt track. On aching legs I carry on running until I reach the church.

You can't go in there you're evil.

Defying the voices I try the door but to my dismay it is locked.

Lightning streaks across the sky and the thunder rumbles in my ears as I crouch down in the church doorway,
I look up into the angry sky. 'Release me!' I shout, 'release from this fear this bondage.
I stay in the doorway for some time until eventually the rain begins to fall down in slow steady spits.

'Come on Lorraine, let's have you back to the ward.
They've got you now.
Two members of staff walk up to me they take my arms and try to encourage me to a standing position.
'Fuck off,' I say.
'Come on now don't start been aggressive.'
They pull me up and lead me back down the dirt track towards the side entrance of Garton ward. And all the time the voices shout out their anger.
You're good for no one.
You will be punished.
Bitch.
Fuck off!' I shout, fuck off out of my head!'

Back on the ward they drag me to the beanbag room.
'You can shout and scream in here to your heart's content,' says the nurse
I stand with my back against the wall fighting with the voices until to my amazement they gradually fade away to silence

'I'm glad to see you've calmed down .' says a nurse as she walks into the small room.' What on earth was all that fuss about?'
Without waiting for an answer the nurse takes my arms, 'come on, ' she says, 'I'll take you for a bath you're absolutely filthy after running through those wet muddy fields.'
Like a naughty child I'm led to the bathroom. The nurse helps me to bathe and after I have dried myself she hands me a blue jogging suit, 'put this on,' she says.
I'm then led back down the stairs and back to the ward. Exhausted I slump in the corner.
Nancy looks on and sighs,' I don't know what the hell was up with you earlier,' she says 'but there was no need to talk to me like that, I mean fancy telling me to fuck off when all I'd done was try to offer a friendly hand.'

I look away from Nancy unable to explain the situation that I'm in.

Chapter 12

They're five people in the small room, the doctor sits behind his desk at his side sits a lady who had introduced herself to me as Jan I look at the badge pined to her blouse and discover she's a psychiatric social worker. A junior Doctor sits opposite her and my Community nurse and a nurse from the ward sit by the door.

The doctor points to a chair, 'do sit down,' he says.

I stay where I prefer to stand.

'How have you been feeling these last few days?' The Doctor sits back in his chair waiting patiently for my reply but I ignore him and look the other way. There is a long silence.

'Lorraine seems to have settled down a little,' says the nurse at length.

'The doctor seems to scrutinise me over the top of his glasses. 'Are you still hearing voices?' he asks.

I shake my head for it's been a few days now since I heard them.

'Good, good,' says the doctor with a nod of his head, 'you seem to be responding to the medication. He looks at the report on his desk and then turns to the nurse. 'I understand that Lorraine's mood is extremely low,' he says.

'Yes she's very withdrawn and also seems a little afraid.,

The doctor glances down at the report again then looks at me. 'Lorraine we have reached a diagnosis,' he says slowly. 'You are suffering from an illness called manic depression.'

His words mean nothing to me so I walk out of the room taking care not to make eye contact with any of the staff as I know 'they're all out to get me.'

'That was rather rude' says the nurse when she came back to the ward .the doctor wanted to explain more about your illness.

'I'm not ill,' I mutter, 'I'm been punished.'

'You are ill and the sooner you accept than the closer you'll be to getting well.' The nurse takes my hand, 'you're not been punished who would want to punish you, you've done nothing wrong.'

I look away from the nurse unable to believe or put my trust in her.

******

The long days drag by, today is Friday, I hate Fridays it upsets me. I watch some of the other patients as they leave the ward to go home for the weekend. It's visiting time Pete sits by my side, he's been telling me how the girls are. I feel hot tears prick my eyelids when he tells me of the funny things they've said and done. I watch sadly as patients carry overnight bags out of the ward.

Pete senses my sadness and puts his arm around me.

'I have to stay here forever don't I,' I mutter.

'Pete shakes his head slowly, 'no,' he says 'do you think I'd let you stay in here for any longer then you need to.'

At that moment the ward Sister walks up to us, she looks at Pete.

'How would you feel about Lorraine going home on weekend leave?' she asks.

Pete smiles however I notice he hesitates slightly.

'Will she be alright?' he asks.

'Well you can always phone us if anything worries you, or bring her back if you feel she isn't up to it.'

Pete looks across at me and smiles, 'would you like that?' he says 'would you like to come home for the weekend.'

I feel my heart somersaulting at the thought of seeing my babies again. My tears of sadness become tears of joy as I nod my head quickly.

'I'll get your medication ready,' the nurse turns and goes into the office.

I'm going home I'm going to see them again.

The nurse returns from the office and hands Pete my weekend medication, she tells him when I should take my tablets.

I'm going home I'm going home.

Pete puts his arm around me and together we leave the ward.

When I walk through the door the girls are sitting watching the Muppets on the television they look up at me unable to believe their eyes. The Muppet show forgotten they run up to me.

'Mammy Mammy you've come home,' says Cheryl.

Pam is sitting in a chair by the door, 'well that was unexpected wasn't it girls.' She says. She turns to Pete, 'Is she alright now?' she asks with a worried expression on her face.

Pete looks at me, 'you're much better aren't you love,' he says.

I gather my little ones in my arms it seems so long since I have seen them. I hold them to me.

'Mammy's just come home for a little while,' says Pete, 'so I want you all to be good girls.'

'Will you have to go back?' says Lucy.

'Yes but she's home for the whole weekend,' says Pete smiling.

'I'll get going home now,' says Pam. She turns to me at the door, 'now the house is reasonably tidy,' she says, 'so make sure it stays that way.'

Pam bustles out of the house.

Later on that evening Pete and I sit back on the sofa watching happily as Cheryl joyfully up tips her toy-box and Lucy and Sammy get out their paints and paper.

Later on we get the girls to bed.

Read me a story Mammy,' says Cheryl excitedly.

I sit by her bed telling her a story watching as her eyelids begin to droop, before I'd finished the story she is sleeping soundly. I look down at my little girl and my heart melts, she is sucking her thumb and seems to have a little smile on her face. I lie by her side and put my arm around here inhaling the sweet scent from her body.

After giving her one last cuddle I leave the room.

Pete looks up he's watching television, it's a news programme, I sit in the corner of the room trying to look away from the television because I know that the newsreader is sending me bad signals.

Pete looks up, 'are you alright love?' he asked.

I fidget in my chair.

'Try to relax love 'you're at home now.'

 Not been able to stand the television any longer I stand up and retreat to the kitchen.

I close the door and walk to the sink, trying hard to drown out the voice of the news reader I turn on both taps. I realise that I haven't had my tablets so I pick up the bottle from the cupboard on the wall. The name of the hospital is written on the label beneath that are the letters BTCH EXP. I drop the bottle in shock for I know that those letters stand for BITCH EXPERTS, and that the voices were right, I am a bitch.

Pete opens the kitchen door, 'what the hell are you doing' he says looking at the water cascading over the sink and flooding the kitchen floor.

He rushes up to the taps and turns them off.

I burst into tears.

It's okay love, it's okay,' says Pete his voice softening, 'did you forget the taps were turned on.

He picks up the bottle of tablets which are now lying up tipped on the floor puts three of them in his hand and gives them to me with a glass of water.

I shake my head, 'I don't want them,' I mutter.'

'You must,' says Pete.

'No.'

'Come on or I will have to ring an ambulance to take you back to the hospital.'

Reluctantly I put them in my mouth and swallow them.

Chapter 13

Cheryl bounces up and down on our bed, 'Are you getting up Mammy,' she squeals excitedly Daddy says that we might be going to the seaside today.
I sit up in bed the early morning sun filters through the windows Pete come through the door carrying a cup of tea.
'Come on you little scamp,' he says to Cheryl ,'don't bother your mammy.'
'But aren't we going to seaside,' says Cheryl.
Pete turns to me how do you feel about a nice drive out,' he says. 'I thought we could take the kids to the beach it's a lovely day not warm enough to sunbathe in but okay for a day out..'
'Please Mammy please,' says Cheryl.
The thought of leaving the house scares me.
Cheryl waits eagerly for my answer.
Not wanting to disappoint her I nod my head trying to force a smile on my face..

We set off early the roads are very busy, 'I think everyone's had the same idea today,' says Pete as he weaves in and out of the traffic.
'I'm going on the donkeys,' says Cheryl, 'and I'm going to make the biggest sandcastle ever.'
'It'not that warm,' laughs Pete, 'it's still only Spring remember.'
'Mam can we go in the amusements?' says Lucy and Sammy in unison.
'We'll see,' says Pete.

After about forty minutes we reach the small seaside town ,the car park is full so Pete parks the car at the side of the road opposite the market. The kids clamber out of the car
'Are you okay?' asks Pete.
I try to muster a smile as I close the car door.
'There are a lot of people here today,' says Pete, 'it's probably because the caravan park has just reopened.'
With my heart in my mouth I take hold of Cheryl's hand she wants' to run on in front but I won't let her and insist that she stays by my side. Many cars line the roads I try not to look in the car windows. An Irate man honks his car horn and rolls down his window,' you stupid bastard!' he shouts.

I scurry along with my heart in my mouth.

I look ahead a group of people are walking towards us.

'Mammy you're squeezing my hand,' says Cheryl.'

'Stay with me,' I mutter it's not safe.'

'She's alright love,' says Pete 'let her run on in front.'

I ignore him. The sweat runs down my back as the people walk nearer, a man stares at me and I can see the contempt in his eyes, *he knows all about me he hates me.*

A woman's shrill laughter fills the air, she's reading my mind, and she knows I'm afraid *Don't look at her keep walking keep your mind blank that's it they've almost past Don't look up keep walking keep walking......* .

'Mammy, mammy please let me run on in front I won't go on the road, I'll be good I promise.'

'She's quite safe,' says Pete.

I loosen my grasp on Cheryl's hand and to my dismay she scampers off to join her big sisters.

Pete takes her place by my side and throws his arm round my shoulders.

'Do you fancy having a look around the market?' he says.

I think of all the people that will be walking around the market and I look at Pete and shake my head quickly.

'Can't understand,' says Pete, 'you used to love markets.'

I look on in front and to my horror the girls are no longer in sight.'

'My babies, they've gone! I told you,' I scream at Pete, 'I told you it wasn't safe.'

'Don't panic they won't be far away.'

'I run up the road screaming out their names. My legs buckle beneath me and I fall to the ground. Pete runs up to me, people pass by with smirks on their faces.

'Are you alright? Asks a man.

'Yeah she's fine,' says Pete as he helps me to stand up.

'The girls have gone the girls have gone!'

Pete points to an amusement arcade next to a row of shops.

'I bet the little sods are in there,' he says

My head aches as we enter the amusement arcade, we find the girls happily threading coins into a one armed bandit. As I run up to them I notice a young man kicking a slot machine he scowls angrily and spits on the floor as I pass.

Pete reaches my side 'I knew they wouldn't be far away,' he says, 'there was no need to get so upset.'

'They could have been anywhere, anyone could have snatched them.'

'Well they haven't and they're quite safe so let's just enjoy the rest of the day, '

'Can we stay in here a bit Mam?' Asks Sammy.

'No,' I mutter.

'Why not,' says Pete 'you could have a go on the bingo; I'll stay with the kids.'

'I don't want to. I don't like it in here.'

The girls sigh disappointedly.

'But you used to love a game of bingo,' says Pete.

'It's not the same anymore,' I say quietly, 'nothing will ever be the same again.'

Pete looks on puzzled as together we all walk out of the amusement arcade.

The Spring sunshine shines down on me as we walk around the seaside town, I hold tightly on to Pete's arm. Directly in front of us well within view walk the girls.

I keep my eyes peeled tightly on them as we walk.

Presently we come to the beach.

'Oh no,' the tide is in,' says Lucy.

'We can't go beach combing now.'

I breathe a sigh of relief.

We sit on the small strip of sand where the water never reaches.

I look towards the sea, it would be so easy so easy just to get up and step into the water and carry on walking and walking....

'Mammy will you help me make a sandcastle?'

Ashamed of my own thoughts I fill Cheryl's small red bucket with sand.

We stay on the beach for some time before we make the slow walk back to the car.

My mouth feels dry, my head aches and my face feels hot.

'Mammy can I have an ice cream?' asks Cheryl.

We stop at the ice cream-stand, 'I want an ice lolly, 'says Lucy.

Pete turns to me, 'what do you want love?' he says.

'Nothing,' I mutter despite the terrible dryness in my mouth.

I hold tightly on to Pete's hand not looking at anyone, hoping the passing people will be fooled into thinking that we're just an ordinary family having a day out.

At last we reach the car.

'Are you okay love?' asks Pete as he drives along, 'you're been really quiet today'

'Yes,' I mutter.

'Has it been a bit too much for you?'

Pete drives the car slowly and carefully until we reach our home

Thankful that the day has nearly come to an end I walk down the path. Although the sun has gone in my face still feels very hot and has started to burn. I walk up the path with my head down.

We have been in the house for about ten minutes when my mam walks through the door. 'How are you feeling love?' she asks putting her arm around my shoulders.

I heard you'd come home for the weekend.'

Although my mam visited me in the hospital it was nice to see her in my own surroundings.

Pete put on the kettle and made a cup of tea.

'You've caught the sun,' says my mam, 'your face is really burnt I didn't think it was that hot.'

I glance into the mirror above the fireplace my face is red and swollen, 'this is part of the punishment for being a bad mother,'. I mutter.

My mam sighs, 'you're not better yet are you love..' she says.

Pete hands me a cup of tea, 'we're due back at the hospital soon,' he says to my mam 'I think this weekends been a bit much for her.'

'Well I suppose times young yet,' says my mam nodding her head and looking towards me as I sit rocking backwards and forwards in my chair.

'Say goodbye to your Mam,' says Pete 'it's time for her to go back to the hospital '

'But I don't want her to go back,' says Cheryl pulling a pet lip.

'She'll be back again soon,' says Pete, 'so you be a good girl for Pam while I take her. 'Lucy puts her arm around her little sister, 'bye mam,' she says Sam kisses my cheek, hurry up and get better,' she says 'we're sick of going to Pam's.

Trying to hold back my tears I walk to the car.

'Don't get upset,' says Pete, 'as soon as you're better you'll be coming home for good.'

******

Have you seen Lorraine's face?' says the nurse when we get back to the ward.

'She seems to have caught the sun,' says Pete, 'but I can't understand it because it wasn't that hot.'

'The nurse looks at me and nods her head knowingly, 'it's a side effect to the drugs she's on ,' she says, 'they make your skin extra sensitive to the sun.'

'Well you might have told us,' says Pete.

'I didn't think,' smiles the nurse.

Pete sighs and after kissing me on the forehead he leaves the ward.

Chapter 14

The doctor walks around the ward he stops at my seat 'you're getting transferred to Sledmere ward this morning,' he says
I feel the colour drain from my face.
'Sledmere ward will be far more suitable for you, it's quieter, more of a convalescence ward, where you will get more rest '
'I don't want to go.'
'You'll be fine,' says the doctor standing up and walking away.

Two hours later I watch as the nurse clears my locker and packs my bag.
'Don't worry,' she says, it's a good sign that you're been moved to Sledmere ward it means that you're on the road to recovery. The next step from Sledmere ward will be going home''
'I don't want to go there.'
the nurse ignores my protests and walks with me to the end of the dormitory.
'You mean I will be going home one day.'
'Of course you will, you just need to learn to put your trust in us, because we're only trying to make you better.'
'I'm bad aren't I,' I say.
The nurse looks directly at me until her eyes are looking warmly into mine, 'you must get it into your head that you're not a bad person and you're not been punished,' she says gently.
'Are you sure?'
'Absolutely certain,' says the nurse. 'You're suffering from paranoia it's a part of the illness.'
Although I really want to put my trust in the nurse I find it difficult to believe and accept what she is saying is true.

I carry my bag across the field towards Sledmere ward. The nurse walks by my side, 'there's no need to be afraid,' she says 'you will soon settle.'
I cast my mind back over the years and recall myself as a young teenager. I recall the excitement I felt when I really thought I was a famous singer. I think about Alex who I used to sing to, Alex who was confirmed to a wheelchair unable to speak or communicate. As we near Sledmere ward I swallow back the bile in my mouth as I remember what they did to him.

We reach the back entrance to Sledmere ward and I shudder. The nurse opens the door and ushers me inside. She takes me to the office and introduces me to Janet the ward sister and then leaves.

'I'll take you to the day-room,' says Janet smiling.

I follow her along the familiar corridor we stop at the dayroom., Janet opens the door and we walk inside. The room is set out almost as I remember it only a CD player now takes the place of the old fashioned record player. I look toward the corner of the room half expecting to see Alex still sitting in his wheel chair but the space is now empty.

Almost as though it was yesterday I remember the morning when two men walked up to Alex one of them put his hand down Alex's trousers. Strange noise had come from Alex's mouth, one of the men turned to me.

'You do it,' he said. 'he likes you you're his little girlfriend.'

I'd burst into tears and the other man had laughed.

The next morning I walked out of the hospital and didn't return until my recent admission just sixteen years later.

'You seem miles away,' says Janet disturbing my thoughts. She introduces me to the other three people who are sitting in the day-room. A man looks up and half smiles he pats the seat next to him.

'Come and sit near me lass,' he says, 'I could do with a bit of company.'

Clinging on to my cigarette packet I sit next to the man, he has a friendly face and reminds me of my Dad.

'The names Jim,' he says shaking my hand.

'I'm Lorraine,' I mutter taking a cigarette from my packet I hastily light it.

'Are you from Garton ward?' asks Jim.

I nod my head inhaling the cigarette smoke at the same time.

'Aha don't worry lass, it's a good sign when you get transferred here, means you're getting better.'

'That's what the nurse said, but I didn't know that I'd been ill.'

Jim laughs, 'well you must have been or you wouldn't be here,' he says.

'Is this really a hospital?'

'Well you could call it that but they used to call it an asylum.'

'It's nowt but a flaming loonybin ,' chirps up an elderly woman sitting opposite me.'

'Am I mad?' I ask.

'No just a bit sick,' says Jim, 'like we all are,' Jim smiles mischievously, 'even some of the staff are a sandwich short of a picnic' he says.

'It can happen to anyone,' says the women, 'people don't realise but anyone can have a mental breakdown.'

'Aye you're right there lass,' says Jim, 'but like I say Lorraine must be getting better now or they wouldn't have put her on this ward.'

Jim turns and looks at me reassuringly   A man who has been sitting in the corner stands up and turns on the television. I get up from my seat and walk across the room.

'Don't you want to watch a bit of telly with us?' says Jim.

I shake my head quickly and walk out of the door.

'Come on I'll show you where your bed is,' says Janet as she comes out of the office.

. I follow her up the stairs. The dormitory isn't much different to the one on Garton ward. Janet leads me to a bed at the end of a long row. Would you like to unpack your clothes.' she says.

I take my bag and fold up my clothes and place them in the locker

'Now I'll make your bed just this once,' says Janet 'but after today you must make it yourself and it needs to be done every morning as soon as you get out or it.'

Having unpacked my clothes I take my small framed photograph of Lucy. Sammy, and Cheryl, and place it on the top of my locker.

'Are those your children?' asks Janet smiling.

'Yes,' I mutter blinking back tears.'

'Oh they're absolutely gorgeous,' Janet turns to me, 'are you missing them.'

I nod my head.

'Try not to worry because we're going to get you better and then you can go back home to them.' Janet looks at me her kind eyes search my face, 'if you ever want to talk about anything or anything is on your mind just come to me,'she says gently.

'I'm scared, 'I say.

'What are you afraid of would you like to talk about it?'

'Everything, I'm frightened of everything.'

'There's no need to be.'

'Am going to be punished?

'No of course not, you've done nothing wrong,' Janet smiles gently, 'and anyway no one gets punished in here. This is a hospital and you're going to get well.'

'But the voices they said......'

'Do you still hear the voices?'

'No,' I mutter.

'You must just think of the voices has been a part of your illness the same as the strange thoughts you are having now.'

Janet smiles sympathetically she touches my arm. 'Don't worry,' she says 'we'll get you well and then you can go home to those lovely children.'

I look into Janet's eyes and I can see she's genuine and for the first time since my admission to the hospital I slowly begin to feel I can trust someone

Janet and I leave the dormitory and go back down the stairs.

Janet stops by the office door, 'don't forget what I said now will you Lorraine,' she says before going inside.

******

The canteen is filling up with people Jim and I sit drinking our coffee a man is intent on telling all who will listen to him that he is the next messiah.

'Take no notice of him love,' says Jim. 'He's not well his head is full of weird ideas and thoughts.'

I sit back in my chair a great sense of relief washes over me, I too must have been ill just like that poor man he can't be the next messiah, so perhaps I'm not a wicked person after all.

The more I think about this the more everything begins to fall into place.

I turn to Jim, 'I'm not bad.' I say..

Jim looks puzzled, 'I beg your pardon love.'

'I'm not wicked or bad.'

'I didn't say you were lass.'

'I've been sick.'

'Well that's what I told you lass, you must have been or you wouldn't be in this place.' Jim sighs and looks around the canteen. 'The best thing for you to do is get yourself out of here.'

Chapter 15

'I'm going home,' I say as I walk into the office.

The nurse looks up from the desk, 'I don't think that would be wise right now,' she says.

'Look the only thing that is bothering me now is been in this place, I need to be home with my family. As soon as Pete visits tonight I'm going home with him.'

'You seem to have made your mind up,' the nurse looks concerned, 'but I don't think the time is right yet you might feel better, which is good, but you need to rest and recuperate before we can even think about you been discharged.'

'I can rest at home better than I can in here,' I say as I leave the office.

Pete is one of the first visitor's to arrive on the ward I run up to him clutching my bags containing my belongings which I'd hastily packed about an hour ago.

'Take me home Pete,' I plead, 'I'm all ready.'

Pete looks down at my bags puzzled, 'did they tell you that you could go home,' he asks.

At that moment the doctor and the nurse walk up to us.

'I understand you want to go home,' says the doctor.

'Yes,' I'm better now. I need to be home to my babies and like I said to the nurse the only thing bothering me now is been here in hospital,' my words tumble out of my mouth in a rush.

The doctor shakes his head slowly 'We have only just got you established on medication, he says, 'so I it would be for the best if you stayed with us a little while longer, you could so easily relapse. You see Lorraine the illness you've got can never be completely cured only controlled by medication and sometimes it can take years to get your medication right so just go home for the weekend and see how you go on and then we'll work towards your eventual discharge.' The doctor smiles and walks away.

He's trying to trick me I'll never get out of here.

'The doctor's right love,' says Pete soothingly, but don't worry, you seem so much better and you'll be coming home for the weekend in a couple of days.'

He doesn't want me to go home, he hates me,.

'Don't look at me like that love,' says Pete, 'it's for the best, look what happened the last time you signed yourself out of here.'

Pete tries to make conversation with me but I ignore him for the rest of the visiting time. 'I'll see you tomorrow,' he says as he stands up to leave.

Saying nothing I turn away.

All the visitors have left the ward now I sit in the corner clutching my overnight bag.

A nurse looks up and smiles, 'Lorraine,' she says 'would you like to go and unpack your bag.'

'I want to go home,' I mutter.

The nurse shakes her head, 'the time's not right,' she says 'you're not out of the woods yet.'

Frustration boils up in me as I unpack my bag, I wanted to go home so much. My babies smile down at me from the photograph on my locker I pick it up and hold it to me tears roll down my cheeks. I would give anything to be tucking them up in their beds and reading them a story. Not wanting to face anyone I sit on the edge of my bed. 'Come on Lorraine we can't have you sitting up here brooding all on your own.'

I look up a smiling nurse faces me, 'try not to get upset,' she says, 'it won't be long until the weekend.'

'Go away,' I mutter.

'Don't be like that.'

'It's alright for you,' I grumble, 'you can go home to a nice comfortable bed and have decent food on your plate, but I have to stop her in this bloody hole.'

'Stop feeling sorry for yourself you want to think yourself lucky you have weekend leave. There's patients in here that can never go home and never even see their families.'

Feeling slightly ashamed of myself I stand up and leave the dormitory. I suppose the nurse is right at least I will be going home for good one day, which is more than I thought not so very long ago.

******

Over the next two days despite my frustration I try to think positive, and before I know it weekend has arrived. Pete slowly drives the car out of the hospital grounds and on to the main road.

'Put your foot down,' I say.

Pete smiles, 'all in good time,' he says as he carefully drives along.

I glance out of the car window a group of people are standing at a bus-stop they stare at me as we pass I immediately turn away and look down.

'What's wrong love?' asks Pete.

'Nothing,' I mutter.

'You're doing ever so well love,' he says 'but I don't think you're quite hundred percent yet are you.'

I shrug my shoulders and say nothing.

The girls are somewhat subdued when we walk into the house there are sitting on the sofa they don't seem at all excited to see me. The house is like a palace, not a toy on the floor or a speck of dust anywhere.

'Oh you're back,' says Pam 'I'll be on my way then.'

'Don't you want a cup of tea before you go? I ask.

'No I've got to get on and you know I don't like tea very much.'

Pam bustles out of the room.

I turn to my girls, 'don't I get a kiss then?'

One by one and without smiling the girls dutifully peck me on the cheek.

I swallow back a lump in my throat, what's happened to my happy babies.

Later on the girls go to bed without making any protest.

'I'll see you in morning,' I say as I tuck them up.

'Mammy,' says Cheryl as I walk to the door. 'Please don't leave us again.'

At that moment I decide that I'm not going to go back to the hospital on Sunday..

Silently I close the bedroom door and return down the stairs.

'What's matter with the girls, there seem so distant.'

Pete looks on and sighs, 'they've missed you love,' he says'

'I'm not going back on Sunday,' I mutter, 'the girls need me.'

'You have to,' says Pete without looking up 'Remember what the doctor said, you could relapse and that would be terrible when you have come so far.'

'I don't care what you say I'm not going back to that bloody place. The girls obviously aren't happy and__'

'Look it would be even worse for them if you relapsed so I'll not hear any more of it you're going back no matter what.'

'I'm not.'

Pete stands up and flicks on the television.

'You can't force me back.'

Pete shakes his head and walks to the television and turns the volume up.

Knowing it's pointless to protest any longer I slam out of the room and go into the kitchen. Such is my frustration I take a cup and hurl it across the floor.

******

The weekend comes to an end all too quickly and before I know it Sunday evening has arrived.

'Are you going to start getting ready to go back,' says Pete.

'I'm not going anywhere,' I say sullenly.

Pete sighs. 'I'm taking the kids to Pam's now and when I come back I want to see you ready.'

'I'm not getting ready, I'm not going back.'

'You have to,' says Pete exasperated, 'you have no bloody tablets left so you have no choice.'

'It's best you go back mam,' says Lucy, 'then you can get properly better.'

I look into my eldest daughter's face and suddenly she seems so old for her eleven years. She turns to Cheryl and Sam, 'come on,' she says in a matter of fact voice we have to go back to Pam's now.'

I stifle my sobs until the door closes behind them. I then go to my bed -room and throw myself on my bed, and sob until my throat feels hoarse. Suddenly my whole body freezes as once again laughter cackles inside my head.

I stay where I am on the bed overcome with frustration and fear. Presently Pete returns he enters the bed- room, 'come on love,' he says gently, 'don't get too upset the kids are going to be alright and so are you.'

I pull myself up into a sitting position, they're back,' I say slowly.

'Who's back?' says Pete.

I place my head in my hands, 'the voices the voices they're laughing at me.'

Pete sits by my side he takes me in his arms, 'I think we should go back to the hospital now love,' he says.

The laughter grows louder as I reach the car Pete gets in the driving seat and I sit by his side. Pete fastens my seat belt and drives off.

'We'll be back soon,' he says looking worried.

As the car speeds up the road my hand goes to the door handle by my side.

I want to open it, unclip my seat belt and throw myself on to the oncoming traffic but something inside stops me. Feeling like a coward I sit back in my seat.

Finally and much to my relief we reach the hospital with shivering limbs and aching stomach I get out of the car. Pete puts his arm around me and together we walk back to the ward.

'Hello Lorraine how's your weekend been?' says Janet.

I burst into tears.

'Oh dear me not too good then?'

'She seems to be hearing things again,' says Pete.

Janet looks at me, 'is that true Lorraine?'

I nod my head quickly.

'Have you been taking your tablets during the weekend?'

'Yes,' says Pete, 'I watched her take them.'

'Well we can't increase her dosage without the doctor's consent, but first thing in the morning I'll enquire about it.' Janet half smiles at Pete, 'I think it will be best if you go now,' she says, try not to worry too much Lorraine's in good hands.' Janet turns and walks away.

Pete kisses my forehead, 'I'll come back and see you tomorrow night,' he says before he hesitantly leaves the ward.

The day-room is empty. I pace the floor, the laughter's unbearable now.

I walk to the bookcase and frantically start pulling out all the books and hurling them across the floor. When the bookcase is empty of books I pick up a pot plant and with all my might I throw it, then watch as the pot smashes against the wall. Anger boils up in me as the laughter reaches a crescendo. I take the rest of the pot plants from off the window ledge and the bookcase and around the room and throw them against the wall. And all the time the laughter roars inside my head.

I turn around as the day room door opens.

'What the hell have you been doing in here!' shouts the male nurse.

Ignoring him I pick up the last pot plant and crash it against the wall

'You can just pick all that up!' says the nurse.

Spent now, I slump in the armchair and rock backwards and forwards.

The laughter has begun to fade away to a dull chant.

I look at all the mess in the day-room and find it hard to believe what I've just done. Janet walks into the room.

'Lorraine's just kicked off Sister,' says the nurse. Janet looks at me and shakes her head annoyed, 'You can just clean it all up!' she says 'I'll be back in ten minutes so you'd better get on with it.'

I get up from my seat and slowly begin to place the books back in the bookcase whilst the male nurse picks up the plants and the broken pottery. 'I can't understand what got into you Lorraine,' he says with a sigh.

Eventually Janet returns, 'it's time for your medication,' she says, 'and then you can take yourself straight to bed and stay there while morning.' She looks at the broken pottery and tuts, 'don't ever do anything like that again.' With that she turns and walks away.

******

I lie in bed and pull the blankets over my head, the laughter has gone now and the dormitory is empty. I feel like a naughty child who has just been punished for having a tantrum. I lie there and will myself to sleep and pray that I don't wake up in the morning.

Chapter 16

The dormitory stinks of sweat and farts; I woke up about ten minutes ago, Morning birdsong fills my ears mingling with the snores and groans coming from the occupants in the surrounding beds. Unable to lie there any longer I get up, put on my dressing gown, wonder towards the door and steal down the stairs.

'It's far too early for you to be up, 'says a nurse, 'come on lets have you back to bed.'

Daring to ignore her, I reach in my dressing gown pocket for my packet of cigarettes and lighter and enter the smoke room where I sit in the corner.

I light a cigarette inhale deeply then watch the smoke as it curls upwards towards the ceiling. I sit back in my chair I look at the smoke ring that has formed and I think of red Indians smoking their peace pipes. I feel an inner calm, so much different to my frustrations of the previous evening.

The door opens abruptly disturbing my tranquillity, a nurse stands over me with her arms folded, 'I thought I told you to go back to bed,' she says.

I take another drag of my cigarette and shrug my shoulders.

'Just wait until the cleaner comes in she's going to play up hell with you. most of those plants are ruined after your little outburst last night__ and as you well know

Sally the cleaner loved those plants tended to them every day she did__ so I should stay out of her way this morning if I were you.'

'I'm sorry,' I mutter.

'And I should think you are,' the nurse then sits on a chair by the door and lights a cigarette.

You idiot woman.

I sit bolt upright in my chair.

You thought we had gone.

Once again laughter erupts in my head.

'Hey pick that cigarette up,' says the nurse.

I look down at the floor but feel unable to move,

'What are you trying to do burn the place down,' says the nurse as she walks over and retrieves the burning cigarette.

Reckless fool.

'Fuck off leave me alone!'

'I'm not going anywhere,' says the nurse, 'I'm staying right here to keep my eye on you we don't want a repeat performance of last night's behaviour.'

She hates you.

She wants you dead.

'Get out of my head, you're not real, you're not real!' I shout.

The Sister pops her head around the door 'Is everything alright?' she says.

The nurse quickly stubs her cigarette in to the overflowing ashtray 'Yes,' she says looking at me 'but it looks like we're in for a day of it.'

I stay where I am in the smoke room and close my eyes tightly trying not to listen to the voices as they rant and rave inside my head. The smoke room fills up with other inmates bleary eyed they light up their cigarettes.

'God I've had a shocking night.'

'So have I never slept a bloody wink.'

The nurse looks my way and shakes her head, 'I think it's time you were dressed,' she says. 'It won't be long before breakfast.'

I stand up and leave the room; I walk up the corridor towards the back stairs that lead to the dormitory.

Everyone hates you.

Your children despise you.

You're a bad mother.

Evil.

You will pay for your sins.

I put my hands over my ears but I can't block out the voices.

Lady bird lady bird fly away home,

Your house is on fire,

And your children are dead.

My heart pounds as I run towards the back door, to my relief it is open, I go outside open fields stretch out before me.   With every ounce of strength in my body I run across the dew soaked grass. I don't know where I'm running to but I know I must get away

But I can still hear the voice no matter how fast and how hard I run.

I fall to the muddy ground and pick myself up and carry on running, *faster, faster.*

In the distance I can see the church I run towards it and stop when I reach the doorway.

I try the door but to my utter dismay it's locked and the door is barred.

Desperate for sanctuary I slump down in the church doorway and sit with my back against the door.

I look up at the grey sky and long to lose myself in the grey swirling clouds.

The voices all seem to be talking at once, they're having a conversation about me.

She's is truly evil

She's too bad to enter a house of God.

I stand up and bang my repeatedly head against the church door, and eventually the voices are silenced.

I hear my name been called, a nurse walks towards me side and takes my arm,

'Come on Lorraine,' she coaxes,' you're in right state come with me you'll feel much better after a nice bath and then the doctor will be here on his ward round.'

I turn and look towards the church my head aches. 'The doors locked,' I say as tears fall down my cheeks, 'I couldn't get in,' I say. 'This place has been locked for years, its derelict now.' The nurse takes my arm and together we walk back to the ward.

I look back towards the old church and think about all the lost and troubled people that must have once visited it.

******

'I understand you are getting the voices again,' says the doctor.

'Yes,' I mutter, 'and I don't think I can stand it for much longer, you tell me the voices aren't real but there must be they must come from somewhere.   Maybe I'm bad or I could be possessed by spirits.'

The doctor shakes his head and smiles, 'well in that case' he says. 'I must have treated a lot of possessed people in my time. Try not to let your imagination run away with you. You have an illness the same as any other, which given time will respond to the correct drugs. So I'm going to change your medication to fortnightly depot injection, you may be more suited to them then the tablets.'

'Will they take away the voices forever?' I ask.

'It should help. 'That's why I think it will be for the best if we start you on them today. And then if all goes well we will discharge you under the care of a Community psychiatric nurse who will visit your home to give you your injection and offer you support. But you

must learn to accept that you have an illness and that you have done nothing wrong and most of all you are not a bad person.'
Full of trepidation I leave the room.

******

'Just a sharp sting,' says the nurse as she pushes the injection in my bottom.
I feel my muscles stiffen up for a few seconds, my body shakes and I want to be sick.
'That's it all done.'
My face flames as I hitch up my pants and once again I feel like a child that has been punished.

******

A week later I'm discharged from the hospital and put under the care of the Community psychiatric nurse.

Chapter 17

The next few months pass by in a haze of bewilderment. The voices come and go and my life is one of fear and uncertainty, filling my mind with unanswered questions. .

Looking after my children and the running of my home has become increasing difficult. Unable to cope with day to day life, my house is often in a chaotic state, I found it difficult to concentrate for very long on any task I set out to do.

My Mam visits when she can but she has moved house now and it is impossible for her to visit me every day. So she comes every week and I look forward to her company, but although she tries it is difficult for her to fully understand what I'm going through. There were times when my Mam seemed to have a magic wand and could easily diminish any problems I was having. Only now no one not even my Mam can ease my troubled mind and make everything alright again.

I often think back to the times before the voices came, times I had once taken for granted. I wish with all my heart that those times would return. But I know deep down that nothing will ever be the same again.

******

This morning is particularly bad the voices are both threatening and under minding. I just can't manage at all, the girls have to get themselves ready for school whilst I sit and stare into space completely immobilised.

'Oh mam you haven't got my P.E kit ready' says Lucy. 'I'm going to be in for it.'

Annoyed and frustrated Lucy slams out of the house.

Cheryl kisses me before she leaves for school. 'see you tonight Mammy,' she says.

Sammy takes her hand and together they leave the house.

The morning passes and the voices fade to a dull mutter.

I sit in my chair, feeling ashamed I look round the untidy room; there is a pile of dirty washing by the cluttered sideboard, and cobwebs hang in the corners. A mixture of toys and books litter the floor and the overflowing ashtrays spill out on to the grubby carpet.

I know I must tidy up but I don't know where to start so I sit back in my chair feeling like a failure.

I look towards the mantelpiece Pete has left a ten pound note behind the clock for me to go to the corner shop to get a bread loaf and something for tea. I know I have to go to the shop as we have no food in the house but the thought of going fills me with dread. Forcing myself I stand up and put on my jacket and take the money from the mantelpiece.

Doesn't she think she's good with ten pounds in her pocket.

I immediately put the money back.

Cheapskate she hasn't got any money.

The voices laugh contemptuously.

I sit back in my chair not knowing what to do for best.

The door bell suddenly rings; hesitantly I go and answer it.

I open the door just a little.

A middle aged women is standing on our step, she has a familiar face but I can't place where I've seen her before.

She looks me up and down. 'I'm the school nurse,' say says, 'and I've come to have a talk with you about your daughter Cheryl, may I come in.'

I open the door wider and the nurse bustles in, she follows me into the living room, but there is nowhere for her to sit as the sofa is full of clothes and old newspapers.

So she stands at the doorway wrinkling her nose and shaking her head. She looks at me with distaste,

'It seems,' she says 'that Cheryl has become a matter of concern her clothes are often dirty and she sometimes smells.'

I feel my cheeks flame with shame.

'The nurse looks around my room, 'now can you make sure she wears clean clothes everyday and has a wash or we may have to contact social services to address the problem.'

.My eyes fill with tears and guilt gnaws at my heart.

When the nurse leaves I pace the floor, *the voices are right I'm a bad mother my child is suffering from neglect.*

I walk into the kitchen the bottles of painkillers are on the top shelf just above the sink. Standing on tiptoe I reach then down and without thinking I open them and cram them all into my mouth, *I'm a bad mother, I'm a bad mother I deserve to die.*

I then imagine my children coming home and finding me dead so in a panic I run to the phone and call Pam.

The phone cackles in my ear presently I hear Pam's voice on the other end of the line.

'Hello.'

'Pam is that you, can you come round?'

'Why, what's wrong now?'

'I need to speak to someone.'

'Are you lonely?'

'I'm having a bad day, I can't cope can you come down.'

'Oh it's just your nerves, get on with your house work there's nothing better for your nerves then doing housework.'

'Can you come down, I'm scared.'

'What are you afraid of?'

'I'm going to die soon.'

'Don't be so stupid it's just your nerves like I keep telling you. So just pull yourself together and get on with........'

'I've took some tablets.'

'What tablets?'

'I've taken an overdose.'

'An overdose you silly, silly girl.'

You're so wretched
The telephone lines are bugged
Everyone knows how foolhardy you are.
Your pathetic voice has been broadcast all over the world.

With my head down and the voices running around inside my head I pace the floor.

Eventually Pam enters the room, she goes into the kitchen and picks up the empty tablet bottle.

'Come on,' she says, 'I'd better take you to hospital

Pam leads me to her car, 'we'll get you sorted out and back to those children,' she says. 'I hope you know they will probably give you a stomach pump, they say it's a horrible experience,' Pam sighs, 'but at least it might put you off doing anything so stupid again.' She mutters.

It seems like all eyes are on us as we enter the casualty department. Taking my arm Pam walks me across to the receptionist's desk. 'She's overdosed on pain killers,' she flusters.

The receptionist looks up, 'if you would like to take a seat,' she says ' I will make sure she is seen next.'

Five minutes later my name is called my legs feel like jelly as I'm taken into a side cubicle.

'Do you remember how long ago it was since you took the tablets?' says the Doctor.

I shrug my shoulders.

'Please try to help me and then I know how to treat you.'

'I think it was about an hour ago,' I falter.

'Why did you take them?'

'Because, I'm a bad mother.'

'What makes you think that?'

I stare at the wall.

My stomach churns and my head feels light   I hear the doctor muttering to the nurse but I can't make out what is been said. The doctor leaves the room and the nurse walks over and stands by my side.

'The doctor has decided that we are to give you an emetic and then admit you for observation,' she says. In the morning you will be transferred to the psychiatric hospital for a little rest. So try not to worry Lorraine, you will feel better soon.'

The door opens, someone comes in carrying a large jug of orange juice and several plastic cups. She places the cups and the juice on to the bedside table.

'Now Lorraine we want you to drink as much juice as you can,' says the nurse.

The cups are then filled with the juice and the nurse hands me each one. I think of Pete and my babies and slowly do as she says. She then gives me a small beaker containing a black tarry looking substance. 'Close your eyes and drink it all down in one go.' The nurse places a sick bowl by my side.

I swallow back the foul looking liquid.

 I feel my stomach reach and I'm overcome with waves of nausea, my whole body trembles as I violently throw up.'

Good girl,' says the nurse,' when I don't think I can be sick anymore ' that's it 'get it all out of your system.'

My stomach feels like cotton wool, exhausted I slump back on to the pillow

'I leave you to rest,' says the nurse as she walks away with the sick bowl.
,
The voices have gone now and I'm still alive. I close my eyes not knowing whether to laugh or cry.

Chapter 18

'Bloody hell lass you're in and out of here like a yoyo,' says Nancy.
We sit in the day room I have just been readmitted to the psychiatric
hospital and I'm back on Garton ward..
'But that's what they always say, "once a patient always a patient,'
'Aye that's true is that Nancy,' says a man in the corner, 'I've lost
count of the number of times I've been brought back to this bloody
place.'
'You will probably keep you in longer this time to make sure you're
properly better before they send you home.' Nancy looks down at
the plastic name bracelet on my wrist, 'oh I see you've been in the
general,' she says, 'what was you doing in there?'
I look away from Nancy, 'don't want to talk about it,' I mutter.
'Did you do something silly?'
I nod my head.
Nancy pats my arm, 'you're in the right place lass,' she says
sympathetically 'there'll get you right eventually.'
'Have they put you on a section,' said the man in the corner.
'No I don't think so .'
'Well they will do if you keep nattering to go home before your
ready,' says Nancy. ' That's what happened to me but my section
ends in a couple of weeks so I may be able to leave then.'
'I'm on a section,' says the man, 'kept escaping I was in hell of a
state when I first came in thought everyone was trying to kill me. It
was a long time before I realised I was ill.' The man looks at me
closely, 'but once you do, you're half way there to getting better.'
'Do you still hear those voices Lorraine?' asks Nancy.
I nod my head quickly.
'You must ignore them or just learn to live with them,' says the
man.'
'Did you get them?' I ask.
'Aye I did, I still do at times but they're not as bad nowadays not
quite as frightening.'
'You've probably got used to them,'
'Perhaps so Nancy, but like I say you learn to live with them.'

I stayed in the day-room for the rest of the morning; I discovered the
man's name was Maurice. As I listened to him talk I slowly began

to realise that I wasn't the only one suffering with this appalling condition. Knowing I wasn't so alone made me feel a little better.

Over the next few weeks I try to settle down into the routine of the hospital life. This is difficult though as all I can think of are my babies. It's visiting time and   Pete has brought them to see me, but the atmosphere is strained, Lucy seems like a different child she is wearing a black leather biker's jacket which she has saved up for and bought herself. It's far too old for her thirteen years but I keep my thoughts to myself.

She faces me across the table, 'when are you coming home Mam,' she asks.

'As soon as she's well enough,' says Pete, 'don't upset your Mam.'

'Well I'm sick of living with Pam, she won't let me even wear lipstick or anything.'

'I'm fed up as well,' mutters Sam I just want you to come home again Mam.'

Pete coughs, 'Pam thought it would be for the best if the girls stayed with her until you're better.'

'Won't let me play with me toys,' says Cheryl, her face then breaks into a smile, 'but sometimes she gives me a Coneto ice cream '

'That's just to stop you nattering,' laughs Lucy, 'and anyway there are making you fat.'

'Well,' says Cheryl pulling out her tongue 'Pam said that if I go to Sunday school I will be able to wear a nice white dress and have my photograph taken.'

Pete went to the toilet and Lucy then informs me in a quiet and grown up voice that she had started her periods that morning. This saddens   me and increases my guilt for I feel I should have been there for her.

 Visiting time comes to an end I watch as the girls follow Pete down the ward, tears splash on to my cheeks as I feel almost as though I 'm slowly losing them.

'Don't get upset lass,' says Nancy, 'you've got a lovely little family and you'll see them again soon.'

'Nothing's ever going to be the same again,' I say in between drags of my cigarette.

Nancy sighs, 'nothing ever is,' she says, 'not when you've had a breakdown. But it seems like you have a good man and he's sticking by you.'

'I want to go home,' I mutter, 'before I lose them.'

'I don't think that will be wise right now,' says Nancy, 'best to stay here love until you're properly better.'

You guttersnipe, your kids hate you.

I stand up and walk away from Nancy but I can't escape from the voice's inside my head. And I know that even if I go home the voices will still be there, so I bite down hard on my bottom lip and try to convince myself that the voices aren't real.

'Your medication has been changed,' says the nurse as she stands by the drug trolley.

'The new doctor had decided to take you off the depot injection as he seems to think you may respond better to a drug called lithium 'You just need to have a blood test taken occasionally to make sure you're on the correct dosage.' The nurse hands me two white tablets and watches me put them in my mouth and swallow them down with water. Feeling somewhat like a guinea pig I sit down.

******

I have been on my new medication for three months now and the voices have gone however I dare not hold my breath and I live in fear of them returning.

I have just been home for the weekend and next weekend. I'm getting discharged for good, I hope and pray that this time everything goes well.

Chapter 19

Eighteen months later.

The coach is coming in just one hour.
I sit up in bed Pete is sleeping by my side.
Get up, get up and be ready.
I get out of bed as quickly and quietly as I can.
You have to be ready for the coach for you are the chosen one.
I enter my living room with the voice running round and round inside my head.
You're going to a party, a special party.
I sit in the armchair, excitement surges through me.
Everyone is waiting for you.
Everyone wants to hear you sing.
You're going to be famous.
I sit on the edge of my seat.
You have the voice of an angel.
I take a cigarette from my packet place it between my lips and pick up my lighter.
 Don't smoke, we can't have that on the coach.
I place the cigarette back in the packet.
Throw them away.
Obeying the voices I quickly throw the cigarettes in the bin.
The coach is coming in fifty minutes.
I steal back up the stairs and go into the bathroom, where I quickly wash my hands and face. I go into my bedroom been careful not to wake Pete I take my best dress from the hanger, and put it on and on tiptoe go back down the stairs.
Brush your hair it's a disgrace, we can't have that on the coach.
I pick up the hair brush and proceed to brush my short thin wispy hair.
Brush it two hundred times.
I look into the mirror and count each brush stroke I make. My arm aches and my scalp is sore after the hundredth stroke I lay the brush down.
I said two hundred times.
I pick the brush back up and frantically brush my hair exactly another hundred times.
The coach is coming in thirty minutes.

You must be ready.
I retrieve my cosmetics from my handbag and for the first time in ages I make myself up.
You need more lipstick, you must look your best for the coach.
I quickly apply more lipstick. My make up applied I turn on the radio, Much to my delight David Bowie is singing one of my favourite songs. *There's a star man waiting in the sky he'd love to come and meet you.......'*
I start dancing around the room and at the top of my voice I sing along to the music.
The door opens and Pete walks into the room he walks up to the radio and turns the volume down.
'What the hell do you think you're doing its three thirty in the bloody morning for gods sake.'
I jump up and down hugging myself with excitement 'did you hear him David Bowie is getting through to me in his songs isn't that great.'
'I don't know what the bloody hell you're going on about Lorraine and why are you wearing all that lipstick you look like a bloody clown with all that slap on your face.'
'Don't you understand I'm going to be famous I can sing I've a got a wonderful voice and I will go far.
'Who told you that? asks Pete.
'The voices, and they're real.'
Pete shakes his head, 'oh no not again,' he mutters half to himself.
'I'm going to a party.'
'No there is no party it's just your imagination.'
The coach is coming in twenty minutes.
The coach is coming to pick me up we're going on tour.
'Lorraine the voices aren't real your getting sick again.'
'I've never being sick you're just trying to trick me again, but I know the voices do exist for I am the chosen one.'
With a troubled look on his face Pete leaves the room.
I open the living room door Pete is standing in the hallway with the telephone receiver held in his hands, he is talking in a hushed tone. Presently he places the recover back in its cradle. 'That was the doctor love,' he says 'he's sending an ambulance, you're not well again.'
'The coach is coming, the coach is coming I don't need no ambulance I'm not sick!'

Pete puts his finger to his lips, Okay just don't wake the girls you go and sit and wait for the coach, it will be here soon,'

'I'll be back in the morning,' I say 'and then we will all go to Disney land on the coach.'

Pete nods his head, 'I know it's going to be great.'

'Is that why you're crying Pete? Are you happy about going to Disney Land?'

'Yes love I am but you must sit quiet and wait.'

I sit back on the armchair I can feel the excitement running through my veins.

The coach will be here in ten minutes.

Pete goes back up the stairs and returns with my small suitcase.

'Is everything ready?' I ask.

'It is, just you sit quiet and wait,

'Have you packed my best clothes?'

Yes love everything is there for you.

The coach will be here in five minutes.

I stand up stand and look in the mirror, 'Pete do I look alright?

Pete smiles, 'you look lovely.'

Someone is knocking on the living room door. A uniformed man enters I run up to him and shake his hand. 'Is the coach here?' I ask unable to keep the excitement from my voice.

The man looks across at Pete, 'Is this Lorraine,' he asks gently.

The coach is waiting for you.

Pete takes me arm and walks with me up the path towards the waiting ambulance, and the voices erupt into laughter.

Where is the coach?

This is the coach, it's a special coach just for you. So hop inside you're going to paradise.

Confused I step into the waiting ambulance. The uniformed man straps me in my seat and we're on our way.

Close your eyes and empty your mind.

Obeying the voices I close my eyes tightly.

Are you tired?' asks the man.

I ignore him and try not to think about anything. A warm wave washes over my body filling me with an inner peace, I feel myself falling to sleep.

'Wake up love, we're here.'

I open my eyes the ambulance has stopped, the door is opened and I'm helped to my feet. Excited I step outside. The familiar large Victorian building faces me.

'Where is everyone,' I ask, what about the party.

The uniformed man looks perplexed, 'party?' he asks, 'there is no party here love you're at the hospital you've come to get well.'

I burst into tears of disappointment and frustration, as I realise that the voices have cruelly deceived me.

Once again I'm admitted to Garton ward.

I go into the smoke-room and much to my dismay I remember that I have thrown my cigarettes away.

A nurse walks into the room I vaguely recognise her.

'Oh it's you back,' she says she looks me up and down, 'haven't you put weight on.'

I sigh for the nurse is right my weight has increased rapidly since my last admittance my doctor says it's a side effect to the tablets I've been taking.

The nurse looks at her watch, 'it's still very early,' she says,' the others won't be up for at least another couple of hours, so why don't you go to bed, I bet you haven't had any sleep all night have you?' Come on I'll take you to your bed.

The nurse jingles a bunch of keys and I follow her as she walks to the dormitory.

My bed is in the corner, 'get yourself laid down and try and get some sleep,' the nurse turns and we'll have a chat later. I sit on the edge of the bed and the nurse turns and walks away.

You've failed the test, you're bad.
You've left your children and your man so alone.
There was never anything planned for you.
It was just a test.
You are not the chosen one.
You've going to burn in hell woman.
Ladybird, ladybird fly away home,
Your house is on fire,
And your children are dead.

With the voices running round in my head I stand up and run to the door.

I leave the dormitory and run down the stairs I can feel my heart beating rapidly. I run down the corridor. Almost out of breath I reach the main entrance. I turn the door handle but it is locked.

'Where do you think you're going? I thought I'd just put you to bed,' says the nurse.

'Home!' I sob, 'I'm going home to my family,

The nurse laughs, 'you'll have job,' she says. 'You're a long way from home.'

Frantic I run up and down the corridor, 'I want to go home!' I shout. 'I'm not staying here.

Changed your tune now haven't you, hiss the voices.

You couldn't wait to get away when you thought you were special.

You're no one, and you're not going anywhere.

You're bad.

'Leave me alone!'

'Be quiet Lorraine,' says the nurse, 'people are still sleeping.'

'Go away!'

The nurse walks over to me and takes my arm and leads me into the smoke-room.

'What's all the bloody commotion about,' she says, 'now sit yourself down and stop making all that fuss.'

'I want to go home.'

'Sit down,' says the nurse 'and as soon as the doctor comes on to the ward I will ask him. But you will have to calm down or he won't let you go anywhere and may even decide to section you.' The nurse shakes her head and leaves the room.

Reluctantly I sit down by the coffee table. I notice a large tab end in the overflowing ash tray I pick it up and place it between my lips. Then disgusted with myself I throw it back down.

Chapter 20

I have been back in the hospital for three months now and in that time I've watched people come and go. I've seen the return of many old faces, one of them is Nancy, but she seemed different somehow, more subdued and not so eager to offer her well meaning advice. She didn't seem to know me when she was first readmitted and it was some time before she would even speak to me.

The doctor has increased my lithium and I now get good and bad days.
On a bad day I'm woken up by the raging voices inside my head and nothing I do will make them go away, however I'm beginning to learn how to ignore them.
I do this by diverting my attention to something else I often count things, I know exactly how many grey tiles there are in the bathroom.
.On a good day I'm woken up to birdsong, like this morning the sun shines through the dormitory windows I feel lighter somehow, like a weight has been taken from my shoulders.
Before I open my eyes I know that today will be a good day.
I sit up and get out of bed quickly and make my way to the bathroom, where I spend some time indulging in a leisurely bath. Then having dressed I make my way down the stairs, none of the other patients are up yet and the ward is reasonably quite.
I walk down the corridor towards the patients telephone pick up the receiver and dial home. After several rings I hear Pete's voice on the other end of the line.
'Hello who is this,' he says tiredly.
'It's me Lorraine.
'Hiya love it's a bit early isn't it are you alright?'
'I'm feeling good in fact I'm thinking about coming home today.'
There's a long pause at the end of the line.
'Pete did you hear me I feel so much better, it's time I was home now with you and the girls, so can you come for me soon,' I say in a rush.'
'Have you spoken to the doctor about it?'
'No not yet but I will soon, Oh Pete I feel so much better, I just know the doctor will let me come home, I miss you so much, but

not to worry because tonight I'll be tucking the girls back up in bed, oh I just can't wait I_ '

'Steady on love,' says Pete in voice that seems to be coming from a long way, 'it's only early days yet The doctor might not agree to you coming home just yet so don't go getting your hopes built up.'

My heart sinks as I hold the receiver tightly to my ear. 'Don't you want me to come back home.'

'Of course I do, it's just that I want you home properly better.'

'But I am I feel so different now.'

I hear Pete sigh the way he does when he's irritated, 'the thing is love' he says, 'I can't have you coming home for just a short while and then having a relapse and having to go back,. It's no good for the kids it unsettles them it will be much better if you wait until you've been well for some time. '

'I'm better and I'm coming home whether you like it or not,' I say into the phone before slamming down the receiver.

I pick up the telephone directory and quickly thumb through the yellow pages until I reach the telephone numbers for the local taxi firms. I choose one and quickly dial the number.

I've been standing outside the front entrance of the hospital for about twenty minutes now.

The taxi should be here soon and I will be on my way home to my babies. I'm so happy to be going home at long last, Pete might be a little annoyed, but when he sees how well I am I know he will also be pleased I'm home.

I look up the road, there isn't many cars just a steady flow of early morning traffic.

Ordinary people enjoying ordinary just like I'm going to do.

Every car I see I pray that it's the taxi but much to my disappointment they all speed by me.

The time passes and I silently pray that the taxi will hurry up.

I hear someone behind me I turn round two nurses face me.

'Lorraine what do you think you're doing out here on the main road.'

'Go away I'm waiting for my taxi, I'm going home.'

The two nurses look at each other.

'I know the taxi firm has rang up its going to be a little late so don't you think you would be better waiting for it on the ward?'

I shake my head and stay where I am.

'Come on you can't wait here all morning.'

The nurses then walk up to me and take me by the arms,

Knowing it's pointless to struggle   I walk with them back to the ward.

'We're calling the doctor,' says the nurse.   'We can't have you leaving the hospital like that.'

The doctors' eyes search my face, 'I've decided that it will be in your best interests if I put you on a section,' he says.

'You can't do that I'm better now and I'm going home.'

'I would rather wait until you have been well a little longer before I even think about your discharge, so try not to get too upset I'm only sectioning you for seventy two hours and then I will see you again and decide on what to do.'

Holding back my tears I leave the consultant room.'

******

'Three days isn't long love,' says Pete.'

'I know but I want to come home now I feel so much better.'

'Give it time love, your only just getting better.'

'Lucy sighs. 'I'd rather you didn't come home if you're not well yet,' she says.

I look at my first born child she seems so old for her fourteen and half years,   and I can't help but feel that she is growing   little detached from me.

Guilt gnaws at my heart for I feel she's missing out on her childhood.

The bell goes signalling the end of visiting time, Pete ruffles my hair and kisses my forehead 'see you tomorrow love,' he says, 'best get back to the other two.'

Lucy gives me a dutiful peck on the cheek.

I watch as she slowly walks to the end of the ward, I wait expecting her to turn and wave to me but she doesn't and just walks out of the door.

During the next three days I feel like a prisoner, the staff observe my every movement and I'm not allowed to leave the ward.   I sit in a chair by the consulting room waiting for the doctor to arrive, I desperately try to compose myself.   However inside I'm very worried, *what if he extends my section, what if I don't go home for month's maybe years.'*

'The doctor is ready for you now,' says the nurse interrupting my thoughts.

Trying to appear confident I walk into the room.

The doctor sits behind his desk, 'and how are you this morning,' he asks.

I try to smile and hope he doesn't see the beads of sweat that runs down my face, 'I'm so much better now..'

The doctor chews the ends of his spectacles, is there anything at all that's bothering you, have you got anything on your mind that you'd like to talk about?.'

There is a short silence and my stomach aches.

The doctor looks up and smiles as he awaits my reply.

I nod my head slowly.

'Would you like to talk about it?

'The only thing that is bothering me now is been here,' I say, 'I know this was the best place for me when I was ill but I feel so much better now. And I need to be home with my family, that's why I rang the taxi the other day I...I.. miss then so much,'

'I understand,' says the doctor, 'but Rome wasn't built in a day you know, so I think we will start you on weekend leave again and see how that goes, I will remove your section in the understanding that you don't try to go home again without permission.'

Knowing I have little choice I agree to this and leave the room.

And so the whole rigmarole of weekend leave starts up again. After my second successful weekend at home I am discharged from the hospital. It's difficult at first but I gradually find myself falling into a routine, and life goes on.

Chapter 21

One year later

I'm filled with a sense of unbearable sadness which has crept on to me like a dark cloud. I can hardly eat and sleep doesn't come easy.. Mornings are the worst I feel I can't face the day. So I stay in bed long after Pete has left for work. Most days I don't bother getting dressed and stay in my unwashed state all week.

My community psychiatric nurse visits once a fortnight she tells me I'm suffering from depression and gives me another relaxation tape to listen to. But it doesn't help as .I find it difficult to concentrate and can't imagine myself walking down a leafy lane when winter fills my heart. My nurse is due to see me today the last time I saw her she said that she was going to get me an early appointment to see the doctor as she feels my medication may need changing. The girls left for school some time ago they left the house before I felt I could force myself out of bed.

Filled with guilt I wonder into the kitchen. There is a trail of cornflakes leading from the cupboard to the sink. A mixture of spilt milk and sugar is stuck to the work surface; and as usual the sink is overflowing with dirty pots. With a sigh I close the door behind me and walk back into the living room. I sit among the debris in my dirty dressing gown and light a cigarette. Suddenly the unwelcome ringing of the doorbell fills my ears. I ignore it hoping that the caller will give up and go away.

Someone tries my door. 'Are you in Lorraine?' Startled I look into my hallway my nurse stands there smiling. 'Oh there you are,' she says brightly. She walks into my living room and moves some magazines and dirty washing and making a space to sit on the sofa. I sit by the unlit fire and fix my gaze on a focus point in the corner of the room.

My nurse takes her large black appointment diary out of her brief case.' 'Would you like to tell me how you feel today?' she asks as she takes in my dirty dressing gown and filthy bare feet..
Her words are met with silence.

'Don't you feel like talking to me?' she says at length. She looks around the untidy living room. I can see you're still not coping very well,' she says.

'I don't know where to start,' I mutter half to my self.

'Well why don't you just set yourself little jobs and begin by cleaning up one room a day.'

I sigh deeply for my nurse doesn't seem to understand how enormous this task seems to me, as I have no energy and don't feel I can concentrate long enough to do anything With an air of efficiency my nurse opens her appointment diary and flicks through the pages. 'I've had a word with the doctor and arranged for him to come and see you this afternoon at two thirty,' she looks at me closely 'he feels that you would greatly benefit from a course of *E.C.T. He says it will lift your mood. She closes her diary and places it back in her brief case and stands up. 'I will be back with the doctor this afternoon and we will be able to discuss this possibility,' she says as she leaves the room.

******

I slowly pack my clothes for my stay in the hospital. I saw the doctor earlier and he wants to admit me this morning to begin a course of E.C.T.

My stomach is in tight knots at the thought of having volts of electric passed through my brain. However my feelings of despair and desperation outweigh my fear of this strange treatment. And the doctor says that there is a good chance of it working and I can then go on to live a normal life.

I'm glad the girls have gone to school for I know I just couldn't bear them to see me leave. We told them that I was going for a little rest the two youngest seemed to accept this but Lucy had looked at me with a strange look on her face and seemed a little surly.

As I finish packing my case I sense that someone is watching me. I turn around Lucy is standing by the bedroom door.

'I thought you'd gone to school,' I say surprised to see her.

'I came back for my P.E kit.' Lucy stands watching me her bottom lip quivers.

'What's wrong love?' I ask.

Lucy breaks down in floods of tears, 'I know what they're going to do to you Mam,' she says in between sobs. 'I overheard you and

my Dad talking saying something about you having electric shock treatment, and I don't want you to have it done. it sounds scary.'
'Your Mam's going to be alright love,' says Pete coming into the room. 'The doctor says the treatment will do her good.
Lucy looks away and I can tell she isn't convinced. She sighs as though she has all the worries of the world on her young shoulders.

Over come with guilt I close my case.

******

 Pete is quiet on the long drive to the hospital and I'm also at a loss for words. I close my eyes and pretend to be sleeping. Finally the car stops Pete taps me on the shoulder.
'We're here love,' he says.
Hesitantly I unclip my seat belt and get out of the car.
Pete takes my case from the boot and together we leave the hospital car park. I feel numb inside as we walk towards the hospital building.

We have been told to go straight to Newland ward as like many other wards Garton ward has now been closed down to make way for Care in the Community.   Eventually all the wards will be closed down and the old Victorian hospital will be pulled down. Patients will then be admitted to the new mental health units nearer to where they live. I have mixed feelings over this new venture as the hospital is the only home some of the longer term patients know. And I feel it will increase homelessness.
We find our way to Newland ward through a maze of corridors, a nurse meets us at the door, she takes us to a room and fills out an admission form and once again I am a patient of Delapole Hospital. The formalities done Pete stands up   'I'll get going now love,' .he says
I walk with him to the door. 'I'll visit you tomorrow night and try not to worry,' Pete kisses my cheek and leaves the ward.

Feeling empty inside I find my way to the smoke room where I sit hidden in the corner.
 Some time later a nurse walks into the smoke room.
'Hi Lorraine,' she says as she sits by my side, 'my name is Julie I will be your key nurse during your stay here.'

I light a cigarette and watch as the smoke forms a perfect ring.

Julie has perfectly manicured nails and hasn't a hair out of place and is a wearing a smart crisp white blouse. A black tailored skirt fits nicely around her tiny waist.

I sit there in my size twenty four faded grey jogging suit with dirty nails and unwashed hair and feel terrible.

'Your treatment starts on Wednesday morning,' she says, 'we thought it best if we let you settle in for a couple of days first. You will have your treatment once a week.'

'How long will I be in here?' I ask.

'Well you are having a course of six treatments so I should think about seven weeks or so.'

'I see,' I say quietly with a tremor in my voice.

Julie smiles warmly, 'there's no need to be afraid, you will be a asleep the whole time, you are given an anaesthetic and won't know a thing.

'Is there any side effects to the treatment?'

'Well you might get a slight headache and feel a little drowsy for a couple of hours but it's nothing to worry about.'

'And what exactly will they do.' I ask.

Julie smoothes her skirt, 'They will place electrodes on your temples which will induce a little fit,' she says with a smile, but don't worry I will be with you the whole time.

'And this will get me better?'Julie nods her head, 'yes more than likely,' she says enthusiastically.

******

I haven't had any sleep all night. I look at my watch it reads six thirty in another three hours I will be having my first treatment of E.C.T. Now the time is drawing near I begin to wish I hadn't agreed to this treatment. However if I had refused it the doctor may have put me on a section and then I wouldn't have any choice in the matter anyway. If only I could just place the covers over my head, go to sleep and not wake up again. The old woman in the next bed moans as she turns around, and the stench of excrement fills my nostrils making me feel sick.

Unable to lie in bed any longer I get up dress in the same clothes as I wore yesterday and leave the dormitory.

I go down the stairs and into the dinning- room a nurse is busy getting the tea trolley prepared.

'I'm afraid you can't have anything to eat or drink until after your treatment,' she reminds me. 'So why don't you go back to bed and get another hours sleep it's only early yet anyway.

I stay where I am looking longingly at the tea trolley.

The clinking of cups fills my ears and the nurse hums a little tune as she fills the large milk jug. Unable to stand it any longer I go to the smoke room. I reach in my pocket for my cigs and despite the terrible dryness in my mouth I light one up.

The rain patters on the grey windows I sit in the corner taking huge drags of my cig.

A middle ages woman sits by the door she half smiles at me.

'Couldn't you sleep either love?' she asks.

I shake my head and look down at the floor.

'I didn't think you could I was in the bed opposite you and I could hear you tossing and turning all night long.' The woman sighs, 'they've taken me off my sleeping pills and I can't sleep a bloody wink without them in fact I'm worse now than I was when I first went on the bloody things. I was on them for seven years, got addicted to them I did, they should never have kept me on them for that long.' The woman lowers her voice, 'to be honest,' she says half to herself. 'I don't think the bloody quacks know what they're doing half the bloody time.'

The woman prattles on in the background but I don't feel like talking to her or anyone else. I just want to be alone, alone with my thoughts.

Presently an old man shuffles through the door, coughing and wheezing he sits on the seat opposite me and proceeds to roll himself a cigarette.

'You're a new face,' he says, 'did you come in yesterday?'

I nod my head.

'Well it's not a bad place if you know the ropes, been in here years I have, I'm doing a long stretch this time.'

The woman laughs, 'Take no notice of that silly old bugger he thinks he's in prison.'

The old man coughs and clears his throat a globule of asthmatic phlegm hits the edge of the waste paper bin.

'You dirty old bastard,' God I'm sick of being in this bloody place.'

The woman tuts in disgust and stands up, 'I'll go and get us a cup of tea, do you take milk and sugar?'

'It's okay,' I mutter.

'Don't you want one you'll feel much better when you get a cuppa inside you.'

'I'm not allowed,' I say.

'Oh are you having the treatment?'

Once again I nod my head.

The woman hovers by the door, and I can see the sympathy in her eyes.

'You poor thing,' she says, I'd hate to have to have that done.'

Trembling I light another cigarette I look at the clock on the wall, and say a silent prayer.

The smoke room begins to fill up with people. At nine o clock prompt a nurse walks into the room.

'It's time to go now Lorraine,' she says.

Hesitantly I stand up and follow the nurse into the corridor where we are joined by two more patients and another member of staff. My legs feel like jelly as we leave the ward and make our way to the E.C.T suite.

We wait in the waiting room.

'Try to relax it will all be over in no time,' says the nurse as she sits filing her fingernails.

Eventually my name is called out and I'm taken to the treatment room.

I can feel my heart beating loudly I just want to run but I know there is nowhere to run to.

There are seven people in the room they all look at me as we walk in.

The nurse points to a trolley, 'would you please get on the trolley and remove any jewellery,' she says.

With a lump in my throat I take off my wedding ring.

I'm then asked to lie down.

Two people stand by my feet whilst two more stand at either side of me.

I can feel the sweat pour down my face, mingling with the tears that run down my cheeks. I feel like a trapped animal and I know there is no escape.

'Close your eyes and start counting backwards from ten,' says a male voice.

My head is pounding I look around me I'm sitting in the waiting room. A nurse sits by my side she is offering me a cup of tea.

'How much longer will I be waiting.' I ask.

'It's all done you've had your treatment for this week.' The nurse smiles, 'there you are you see, I told you it would be all over before you knew it, 'you're in recovery.'

I look around me and remember the sterile room the staring faces and I'm overcome by a feeling of fear and unreality.

'Sit and have a little rest and I'll take you back to your ward.'

My teacup shakes as I hold it to my mouth, my stomach churns as I sip the sweet sickly tea. My head throbs as the pain becomes intense.

Chapter 22

My course of E.C.T has now finished.   My head aches constantly
and I feel numb inside. Pete's taking me home in the morning, it's
difficult to tell whether the treatment has worked until I'm back in
my own surroundings faced with the pressures of everyday life.
However I'm relieved that the treatment is over and I will be soon
back home again with my family.
   I lie in bed and pray for sleep to come, anything to release me from
the terrible pain inside my head. I was given two painkillers about
an hour ago but they haven't kicked in yet. I put the covers over my
head until I'm cocooned in darkness.
   The hours pass and I feel myself drift into a light sleep.

'Morning Lorraine,' says a nurse.
I slowly sit up in bed the pain has gone but my head feels numb.
'How do you feel sigh the nurse's chirpy voice grates. 'Cheer up
you're going home this morning.'
It's difficult to get enthusiastic as I don't know if I will be able to
cope once I'm home. Things are so different in the hospital most of
my decisions are made for me and I don't have to think for myself.
I just go through the motions of day to day life. pray that after my
discharge everything will go well, that I won't ever have to return
to this forgotten place.

In a daze I go to the bathroom where I splash cold water on my face,
ever since the electric shock treatments I've felt strange, sort of
detached from reality.
'Why don't you have a nice bath?' says the nurse.I turn around and
shake my head.
'I'm sure you'll feel much better, you should have a bath every
morning.' The nurse runs the water for the bath and pulls the
curtains around it. 'You shouldn't neglect yourself.'
   Gingerly I step into the tepid water.
'Wash yourself all over,' the nurse hands me the bar of green
unscented soap and the grey flannel and leaves the bath room.
I lie there in the bath for some time it will be so easy, I tell myself,
so easy just to put my head under the water and stay there, then I
will no longer be a burden to my family, to myself....

The bathroom door opens the nurse pops her head around the curtain.

'Are you all right Lorraine, you've been in here ages.'

Relieved that my thoughts have been disturbed I stand up quickly and get out of the bath.

Having dried myself I dress and go down the stairs.

'Your husband just phoned,' says the sister 'he's on his way to pick you up.'

Full of mixed feelings I go back to the dormitory and pack my clothes.

******

The girls are at school when Pete and I arrive home from the hospital.

The first thing I do is put the kettle on to make a cup of tea.

'I'm real glad you're home love,' says Pete 'I've really missed you. Pete takes me in his arms, but I can't return his embrace, I feel awkward and detached.

I push him away, 'what's wrong,' says Pete looking hurt and rejected

'Nothing,' I mutter reaching for the cups.

'Are you feeling better now?'

'I'm not sure.'

'What do you mean you're not sure?'

Ignoring Pete I finish making the tea we carry our cups into the living room and sit down. Pete sits by my side on the sofa and I drink my tea in silence.

'You'll soon settle back in,' says Pete at length 'things are bound to be a little strange at first.'

I sigh wishing I could share my husband's enthusiasm.

Chapter 23

Since having E.C.T I have found that my concentration has grown worse. I can't focus on hardly anything, I can't seem to follow a television programme or hold a conversation with anyone as I find that I lose the thread of what I'm talking about.

A lot of early precious memories have been wiped out, I can't recall milestones like my children's first words their first smiles and their first steps.

I find that I have to look at their baby photographs to remind me of what they looked like when there were younger. Pete often talks of incidents which have happened over the years but sadly I can't remember them. I feel like I'm locked in the present with just a faded and broken past. Every day is the same although I try to carry on I find it difficult. I still suffer with severe headaches and they are days when I feel physically as well as mentally unable to cope. As a result my house work suffers badly and however hard I try I don't feel my children are receiving the attention that they need during their growing years.

Pam still takes Sammy and Cheryl to Sunday school each week, She buys them sweets and ice-creams for going. However being that bit older Lucy refuses to be bribed and dyes her hair green instead.

My mam phones me up every day, she tells me not to worry about the house work and concentrate on getting better. Despite being a grown woman I miss her so much as I used to go and visit her every day and was used to being a part of an extended family I know she's only a bus-ride away but I find it difficult to go out.

She comes to see me once a week but things just don't seem the same. She tries to talk to me and tells me that I'm doing well and that it's not my fault that I'm sick.

However I still feel guilty.

******

My girls are all growing Lucy will soon be leaving school and is hoping to get a place at art college. Samantha and Cheryl seem to be doing well. However I worry about them a lot and hope that my illness has not affected them in any way as life can't have been very easy for them.

One year later

Chapter 24

'She's just been a teenager,' says Pete when I discover that Lucy has left home and has gone to live at a hostel in Hull.
'But she is only sixteen,' I mutter with tears pouring down my face.
'Well we can't do anything about it,' says Pete.
'It's my fault,' I say 'perhaps social services feel that I'm not capable of looking after her.'
'It's not your fault at all love, you can't help being ill and you have never hurt or neglected her in any way.'
'But it's all she's seen most of her life me in and out of hospital and_'
'She'll be back, try not to worry she's just been a bit rebellious right now and wants to live with her boyfriend.
However Lucy didn't come home but moved from the hostel into a flat where she lived with her boyfriend. The flat the hostel had found them was in the red light area of Hull. Not a very safe place for vulnerable and impressionable teenagers.
My hands are tied and there is nothing I can do to bring my daughter back home.

Much to my distress I later learn that Lucy has dropped out of Art college and is experiencing serious problems.
With nowhere to turn I speak with the college councillor.
I ask her if she can get in touch with Lucy's key-worker and find out what support my daughter is receiving. The counsellor then rings up the key-worker who is based in Hull. After her telephone conversation which lasts about ten minutes she looks up at me and simply states.' that she can not tell me anything as I'm a manic depressive.'
I walk away feeling like a criminal a lesser person.

Chapter 25

I woke early this morning before the first light. Sitting by the unlit fire I look around the untidy living room, the dirty carpet and the cobwebs in the corners. Sighing I stand up and open the grimy faded curtains and to my surprise I notice that the sun is shining. The clock on the mantelpiece reads six ten. I know Pete and the girls won't be up for some time yet as today is Sunday and there will be having a lie in. An image forms in my mind an image of Pete and the girls getting up to a spotless house and me refreshed and happy cooking them Sunday breakfast. It could be like that, I tell myself *it's all down to you.*

A surge of adrenalin runs through me as I take down the dirty curtains and open the window to let it some fresh air. I scurry into the kitchen and pull the twin tub from under the sink, and fill it with hot water add the detergent and the curtains. I'm filled with a great sense of relief as I turn on the washing machine. With my arms full of dusters, polish and disinfectant I return to the living room. I look down at my carpet and notice how filthy it is I decide that it is well past scrubbing clean so I clear the floor then I begin pulling up the offending carpet. It takes some time as I have to move the furniture and pull it from underneath. I take a Stanley knife and cut the carpet away in squares then I place it all in bin liners and put them by the back door.

Exhausted I look down at my grimy floorboards. I go into the kitchen and return with a bucket full of water detergent and a scrubbing brush. On my hands and knees I begin scrubbing the floorboards.

You slatternly bitch your house is filthy.

I turn quickly and knock over the bucket of water.

You idiot you can't do anything.

Trying to ignore the return of the voices in my head I attempt to mop up the water as it slops on to the floor boards soaking them. However I just seem to make things worse as the water spreads wetting more of the boards.

I look around the room and begin moving ornaments and junk off the cluttered side boards and shelves. I place the ornaments on the sofa one of them falls of and smashes on to the wet floor.

Useless bitch.

Overcome with frustration and with tears raining down my cheeks one by one I snatch up the rest of my ornaments and hurl them across the floor smashing them. And all the time the voices rant and rave inside my head.

Failure.
Foolish cow.
She's bad
She's possessed by the devil
She can't do anything.

Just as I'm throwing the last ornament across the room the door opens.

'What the hells going on?' says Pete 'it looks like a bloody bombs hit it in here.

Pete stares at the broken pieces of pottery on the floor, his face drops. He looks down at the bare floor boards, 'where's the carpet?'

'It was filthy so I pulled it up.'

'My God Lorraine what on earths got into you.

The devil,' I reply, 'I'm possessed by the devil.

'I think you've been overdoing it.' Pete shakes his head and sighs loudly, 'I don't know how we're going to afford a new carpet.'

'Did you hear what I just said? I'm possessed by the devil.'

'Don't start talking a load of shit love especially in front of the kids you'll scare them half to death.'

'But I'm possessed........'

'No you are not,' says Pete shaking his head 'you're just not well again,'

Pete sits on the sofa looking at my collection of Russian nesting dolls that lie smashed and broken in the floor. 'Oh Lorraine,' he says 'you really loved those dolls.'

'I don't deserve nice things I'm bad.'

'No you're not you've been a real good lass so you can get that idea out of your head.'

'The voices tell me I'm bad and I believe them.'

Pete's face drops 'are they back?' he asks.

'Yes and they are real so it's no good trying to tell me otherwise.'

'How can they be when there inside your head no one else can hear them.'

'Because I'm the chosen one, chosen because I'm bad.'

Pete looks exasperated, 'how many times do have to tell you don't listen to the bloody voices, just listen to people you can see. Try listening to me for a change especially when I tell you that the voices are a part of your illness.'

At that moment the door opens Sammy walks into the room, her bottom lip quivers when she sees the smashed ornaments on the floor. 'Mammy have we had a burglar in the night,' she says.

'No Mam was just doing some Spring cleaning and she accidently drooped them. And don't worry about the carpet it was very dirty so Mam pulled it up because we're going to get a nice new one.'

Cheryl walks over to the smashed ornaments and picks up the remains of a shattered porcelain rabbit.

'Oh Mam I bought you this for a present.'

'Never mind, 'maybe you can buy her another one,' says Pete.

Cheryl pulls a pet lip 'I don't want to if she's not going to look after it.'

Pete gets on his hands and knees and begins to pick up my smashed once treasured ornaments.

'Your going to have to get yourself sorted out,' he mutters to me, 'it's not good for the kids it's not good for anyone.'

******

As the day passes the voices become more and more obnoxious and fill my head with their obscene insults and threats. I retreat into a world of my own where I'm not aware of anything but my own paranoid thoughts.

I vaguely remember my Mam coming down she tries to talk me round but I ignore her and retire to my room. I'm too afraid to talk because the voices twist my words and mock everything I say. I sit on the edge of my bed with my head in my hands convinced that I am indeed possessed by a bad spirit.

Pete tries to coax me into coming down the stairs but I stay in the bedroom not wanting to face anyone. The time passes slowly I can hear people talking and laughing outside and I know I'm the subject of their mirth.

I go to the window to close the curtains, *shut them out shut them out shut out the world.* Music floats up to me from the radio downstairs, *I can see clearly now that 'Lorraine' has gone, it's that song again,* I scream silently and the voices laugh and jeer

Chapter 26

I'm sitting in a tiny room with my dressing gown pulled tightly around me. My head feels muggy and my mouth is parched.

'How are you feeling today asks a women sitting by my side, 'you was in a hell of a state when they brought you in you wouldn't stop screaming.'

I cast my mind back images and feelings slowly come back to me, my failed attempt at cleaning the house, the fear and the return of the voices and the persecuting song on the radio. After that my mind is a blank.

'Where am I?' My voice quivers I sound like I'm coming from a long way.

'Your here with us love,' says a man sitting opposite me.

'What am I doing here?'

'You're sick, when they brought you in you were running up the corridor screaming like a banshee, but you have been a lot quieter this last few days a bit strange though. Do you remember thinking that the fire alarms were babies?'

I quickly shake my head.

'Never mind love you're in the right place,'

I look around the small room the place is unfamiliar to me and all I can smell is furniture polish and wet paint.

'Where am I?'

At that moment a young women walks through the door.'

'Have you got my tablets nurse?' says the man.

'I'm not allowed to give you them I'm only a student nurse,'

The man sighs and leaves the room.

The student sits by my side.

'Where am I?' I repeat almost to myself.

'Your in Nidderdale,'

'Nidderdale?'

'Nidderdale mental health unit. The hospital has been closed down, it's Care in the Community now,' says the student with a smile.

'Will I be staying here long?'

'No just until there's a bed for you at Rosedale a unit which is closer to your home.'

'But I've got my Spring cleaning to do.'

'Well I'm sure that can wait_'

'But the voices they told me that I'm a failure, a bad mother I must get it done, I've got to get home to my kids_.'

The student half smiles pats my arm and walks out of the room.

'There always running short of beds in these units,' says a woman in the corner.

'Shouldn't have closed the hospitals down,' that's what I say,'

The woman points to an old man who's sitting by the window, his face is grey and he has a look of fear in his sunken eyes.

'I mean look at poor Jim been a patient at Delapole hospital most of his days only home he's ever really known. He was brought in here last month found him wondering about around Town not knowing where the hell he was. He can't cope on the outside you know.'

'I know but the units are much nicer the food and everything and even the staff seem to treat you better,' says the man sitting opposite me.'

The woman sighs, 'that's when there are enough beds,' she mutters.

I don't say anything as I'm too worried about my future and what will become of me.

The next few days pass by in a haze of confusion and turmoil I feel so afraid. I'm careful who I speak to and I only eat a little as I'm certain that I'm been poisoned.

After yet another restless night. I'm called into the office. A nurse looks up at me as I enter. 'You're getting transferred to Rosedale ' she says 'they have a bed available for you.

Rosedale is in Hedon about a mile away from my house, they say it's the new mental health unit but I know different, I know that when I get there I will be punished I know they're waiting, waiting for me_

A nurse leads me to the waiting car, 'Don't worry you will be a lot better off; You will be right near your home so it will be so much easier for your husband to visit you at Rosedale.' The nurse smiles, 'and you will be in the lap of luxury there because I've heard that Rosedale is one of the best units.'

Slowly I get into the car the nurse gets in the driving seat and straps me in. 'We'll be there before you know it, she says.

I sit in my seat as the car drives through the City I avoid looking out of the window and keep my head down. The nurse tries to keep up a conversation as she drives along but I ignore her because I know that like the others she is out to get me.

Chapter 27

It's been a long night and I haven't slept a wink, daylight has just begun to filter through the curtains, I get out of bed, put on my dressing gown and slippers and leave my room.

Apart from two nurses the office is empty no one notices me as I creep by. I pass the day-room and I can hear snoring. The alarm goes off as I open the door so I quickly step outside closing the door behind me.

The grounds at Rosedale are not as nearly as large as the grounds at Delapole hospital and are more like a large garden. It's a nice spring morning I watch as a squirrel runs up a tree and I envy its freedom.

I stand looking up into the tree and I'm certain that David Bowie is sitting in the top branches waiting for me. Using all my effort I begin to climb the tree, however I can only reach the first branch so I sit there for some time with tears pouring down my cheeks.

A slow steady drizzle comes from the early morning sky as I back climb down.

I walk around the grounds for some time not really caring that I'm slowly getting soaked to the skin. Eventually I return to the unit.. The staff are busy in the office handing over to the day staff. I steal by and go back to my room.

I open my curtains and stand with my face pressed against the window.

I look up into the tree I had just tried to climb but to my dismay there is no-one sitting in the branches.

Having changed out of my soaking wet nightgown I leave my room. I'm greeted by a smiling nurse, 'you've had a good sleep, night staff told me you slept like a log all night.'

******

It's nearing the end of visiting time I walk with Pete to the door. 'You've got to snap out of it love,' he says.'

'I want to go home.'

'But they won't let you love, not until you get well, not until you realise that your mind is playing tricks with you again.'

'They all hate me they're going to kill me because I'm bad don't leave me here.'

'That's just the paranoia,, your imaginations working overtime again.'

'I'm evil.'

Pete sighs, 'I don't know what the hell gives you that idea.'

'I know I am.'

'I suppose the voices tell you. Why don't you stop listening to them you did last time and you got better.'

I turn away from Pete knowing that it is futile to ignore the voices because they always come back with a vengeance. Pete stands at the door waving I watch him as he walks down the path towards the car-park.

'You want to listen to what that husband of yours tells you,' says a man who had been eavesdropping in the background. I ignore him but he walks by my side and he follows me into the smoke room. He sits by my side and offers me a cigarette. 'The names Stan,' he says with a smile

To afraid to accept the cigarette I look away.

'You'll be alright lass,' says Stan with a smile, 'it just takes time that's all it took me years.' Stan stands up, 'when you feel like talking to someone I'm a good listener,' he says   before sitting down a few seats away from me.

The morning passes and the smoke-room fills up with people, some try to involve me in their conversations but I just sit with my head down.

A women sighs, 'she's bloody ignoring us,' she says.

'The poor lass is paranoid,' says Stan,' best to leave her until she comes round.'

The woman gives me a sympathetic look, 'there's nowt worse then paranoia, I've had my share of that I can tell you.'

Stan nods his head in agreement, 'aye I remember Doreen, bloody hell when you first came in you wouldn't even look at anybody never mind talk to them.'

'Best to keep taking the tablets that's what I say they've sorted my head out.'

'You was lucky Doreen,' says a young man as he rolls a cigarette, took them ages to find a drug which suited me, even now I still have me bad days.'

Doreen looks my way, 'don't worry they say everyone gets better in the end.'

With all my heart I want to believe Doreen but I find this difficult as the voices and my strange thoughts seem so real.
However over the next few weeks I find that the more I listen to my fellow patients conversations the more I slowly begin to realise that I am ill again.

Life on the unit is much better than life in Delapole hospital, I have my own room and the food is a great improvement to the disgusting slop that was served out at Delapole.   Visiting time is much easier as the unit is only about a mile away from where I live. And It feels better somehow knowing that I'm not so far away from home.
At Rosedale I feel like a person whereas at Delapole I felt I was just a number.

******

After a further four weeks at Rosedale I am discharged. I'm well for quite some time, until once again I'm stooped into a world of fear where the voices rage and thought delusions take over my mind.
****
Due to stress family relationships have become a little strained over the years.
Cheryl becomes the victim of school bullies which causes her to be very withdrawn and extremely shy. Despite complaining about this the problem is never fully resolved until she leaves school. However by then the damage has been done and Cheryl grows more and more distant.
Lucy splits up with her boyfriend and Sammy moves in with her, I'm not sure when this happened but it isn't long before I discover that Sammy is also having problems.
During the periods that I'm well I begin writing a novel, Only I rip it to shreds each time I become ill. The novel is very important to me as my main character has mental health problems, and   it highlights the stigma attached to this illness. I find writing very therapeutic as it takes my mind off my worries for a short while.

In order to gain confidence I enrol on a creative writing course at Hull College, I find that this helps me a great deal and it offers me the chance to get out of the house and meet people.
However during the course my illness rears its ugly head and my work is reduced to shreds once again.

******

Over the next few years I have many relapses in my mental health which require further admissions to various units. My medication is changed many times and I'm given another course of E.C.T which leaves me disorientated for months.

Sadly after a family argument I lose touch with my firstborn. Sammy moves in with her new boyfriend and seems happy, a few months later Sammy breaks the news that she's going to have a baby. I'm overjoyed at the thought of becoming a grandmother however not a day goes by when I don't think about Lucy and I hope and pray that one day we will all be together again.

Chapter 28

The sky is grey and a drizzle of rain seeps into my skin. Pete and I walk around Hull city centre. We have been to the travel agents to book a holiday to Spain.

We make our way down Whitefriargate which is one of the main shopping areas in the City.

As we walk I begin to get the feeling that Lucy is near it's like I can sense her presence. I stop dead in my tracks.

'What's wrong?' asks Pete.

'It's our Lucy she's here.'

'Where?' Pete scans the crowds of people.

'I just know she's around here.'

Pete looks puzzled,

'How do you know.'

'I just know that's all.'

I then break into a run and start shouting her name at the top of my voice hoping that she'll hear me. People turn and I'm aware of their strange looks a woman laughs, but I don't care I just want to see my baby.

Pete catches up with me and takes my arm, 'come on love,' he says 'Lucy isn't here you're just imagining things again.'

Reluctantly I let Pete lead me to the car-park. As I walk I scan the crowd of shoppers hoping to catch a glimpse of my daughter.

Once inside the car Pete searches my face, 'you're not well are you love,' he says as he starts the engine, 'I can tell by your eyes.'

I sit in the front seat with my face pressed up against the window People scurry by all going different ways all living their own lives.

'You'll see her again one day,' says Pete as he drives along, 'you've just got to let her make her own mistakes, She's a woman now no longer a kid you can't be responsible for her anymore.'

Pete's words do nothing to console me for no matter how old she is Lucy will always be my baby.

We arrive home and I go straight to my bedroom with tears pouring down my face I throw myself on to the bed. Suddenly the familiar chanting of the voices erupt inside my head.

You are a bad mother.

Evil.

Wicked.

Hell is waiting for you.

I pull the blankets over my head but it doesn't drown out the voices. I can feel someone shaking me.

'Go away!' I scream

'Lorraine it's me what's wrong? 'Pete pulls the blankets away.

You're dying

Go away!'

Come on love you don't want to be up here all on your own.

I sit up and place my arms around Pete's neck, 'hold me hold me tight,' I say.

'What's wrong love?'

'I'm scared.'

There's no need to be scared love I'm here.'

You can't die in that mans arms.

You've been together for hundreds of years.

Every life time, since the beginning of time,

But next time it will be different.

He hates you, he hates you.

'Come on love, come and watch a bit of telly or something.'

I push Pete away, 'why do you hate me?' I say.'

Pete looks perplexed, 'I could never hate you,' he says before leaving the room.

I lay back on the bed close my eyes and will the voices to go away.

The hours pass Pete brings me tea but I just leave it by the side as I'm not sure I can trust him anymore.

Later on Pete come to bed I lie as far away from him as I can and stare into the darkness.

Sleep finally releases me from the voices however it seems like I've only been sleeping for a very short time when I'm awakened by the alarm clock ringing insistently in my ear.

'How are you feeling today?' asks Pete the moment he opens his eyes.

I ignore him as I climb out of bed.

'You're not well are you love.'Pete sits up in bed, I think it will be a good idea to ring your C'P.N,' he says.

Saying nothing I leave the room.

About three hours later my C.P.N arrives. Pete brings him into our living room he sits on our sofa staring at me placing his brief case by his side.

'What's matter Lorraine,' he asks at length.

He's laughing at you,' whispers the voices.

I sit opposite my C.P.N trying to avoid his stare.

'Would you like to tell me how you have been feeling?'

'No go away piss off out of my home.'

'Are you hearing voices again?'

He mocks you.

'Look just take your case get off my sofa and leave my home.'

'Lorraine this isn't like you, would you like to talk about what's bothering you.'

'Fuck off!'

My C.P.N. looks on shocked by my out burst. But I'd just had enough and all I want is to be alone. The C.P.N stares at me and there is another short silence as he searchers my face.

'Go on then piss off!' I shout unable to control my anger.

'Okay I'm going,' the C.P.N stands up and walks out of the room. I sit back in my chair I can hear him talking to Pete as he leaves the house but I can't make out what they are saying.

About two hours later my C.P.N returns with a doctor.

'I hear you're not well Lorraine,' the doctor stands by the living room door.

I look the other way refusing to meet the doctor's eyes.

'Are you hearing voices?'

I nod my had slowly.

'Have you been taking your tablets?'

'Yes I always make sure she has them,' says Pete.

Perhaps you need your medication changing how do you feel about going in the unit for a few days?'

My C.P.N turns to the doctor, 'there isn't any beds at Rosedale at the moment,' he says.

It is then arranged that I'm to stay at a unit in Bridlington until a bed becomes available at Rosedale.

Chapter 29

The next few days seem to merge together; I'm not sure where I am for I have never been on this unit before so the place is not familiar to me. All I know is that the strange staring faces belong to the other side ,they despise me and want to do me harm. I know what they are thinking when they stare at me in contempt as I pass.

I see Pete sometimes he seems different somehow, I told him I want to come home but he feels it will be for the best if I stay here. I think he hates me too and I wonder if I'll ever get home again.

I sit in the small crowded room a haze of cigarette smoke fills the air; everyone seems to be talking at once as the radio plays constantly. Earlier I tried to escape to my room but they brought me back as sleeping is not allowed during the day. So I sit here quietly hoping I'm not noticed as I try not to make eye contact with anyone.   A member of staff pokes her head around the door she looks my way, 'Lorraine we would like a word with you in the office,' she says.

Hesitantly and with my head down I stand up and follow her down the corridor and to the small office. A woman smiles when I enter but I know it's false. I shudder as I face the large desk .

'A bed is available for you at Rosedale,' she says with a smile, 'so could you get your things together and wait by the main door and I will take you there in the unit's car.'

I go straight to my room bundle my clothes up in a carrier bag and make my way to the main entrance.

****

My head aches considerably as the nurse drives along.

'We'll be there soon,' she says cheerily.

My thoughts in a whirl I look down at my trembling hands, they're all waiting for me. What are they going to do to me when I get there?

They're going to punish you, cackle the voices.

You are bad,

You are bad.

You will get what you deserve.

The nurse turns on the car radio music plays and the nurse hums away to a tune.

My head throbs all I want to do is get out of the car but I know there is no escape.

I know I must face up to whatever is in store for me.

We reach Rosedale around lunchtime where I'm admitted and taken to the dining- room. Although my stomach grumbles I refuse to touch any of the food that is placed in front of me. Some of the staff have familiar faces which I remember from my other frequent admissions however I don't feel I can put my trust in any of them.

Leaving the dining table behind me I go into the lounge a nurse is placing beanbags on the floor she look up at me as I enter. 'Relaxation will be starting soon,' she says and we like everyone to take part, it's very good for you, She pats a beanbag,' sit yourself down, you might as well wait for the others to join us.'

Feeling as though I have little choice in the matter I sit down.

Presently some of my fellow inmate enter the room and take their places on the beanbags.

The nurse stands and fiddles with a small stereo set and puts on a tape and a haunting tune fills the air.

The nurse begins to talk with a deliberate slowness in her voice as though she's addressing a group of children.

'C l o s e your eyes,' she says, the music tinkles in the background. 'You are going for a walk in a beautiful garden the sun is warm on your back.'

I keep my eyes wide open she is trying to get into your mind I warn myself trying to read your thoughts.

My stomach growls loudly and I can hear the creaking of someone's bones as they stretch out on the beanbag.

'Look at the beautiful flowers a profusion of colour greets you as you walk down the winding path. You can almost smell the sweet perfume and......... .'

Someone farts loudly and I hear the sound of smothered laughter.

Not distracted the nurse drones on and the music plays softly and gently for some time. My mouth feels dry as I desperately try to clear my mind of everything.

After some time the relaxation session comes to an end I sit up and as I leave the room I notice two of my fellow inmates have fallen asleep. The nurse smiles smugly for they are now in her power.

Lying in bed that night I will myself to stay awake feeling that if I fall asleep I will be off my guard and my mind will be taken over by those on the other side

I lie listening in the dark as the church clock strikes away the hours.

At last the clock strikes five o'clock relived I get out of bed and put on my dressing gown. I am filled with an uncontrollable urge to smoke, smoking is not allowed in my room so after placing my cigarettes in my pocket I quietly leave.

The smoke room is empty sighing with relief I place a cigarette between my lips.
As I light it the screeching of the voices erupts inside my head.
Put it out bitch put it out now.
I inhale my first drag of the cigarette.
Put it out something bad will happen if you don't!
Desperate to smoke my cigarette I take another drag and inhale the smoke deeply.
Evil bitch.
Wicked troublesome cow.
Someone in the world will die soon because you ignored us.
In shock I drop the cigarette by my side.
At that moment a nurse walks into the smoke- room
'You'll be the death of us all,' she says crossly as she bends and picks up the lit cigarette which has left yet another small round burnt hole on the grey carpet.
Consumed with guilt I leave the smoke room.
 I sit in the lounge with my head in my hands.
Although the voices have forbidden me to smoke I still want one in fact I feel I need one so badly it is all I can think about.
A cleaner busies herself as wipes imaginary dust from the coffee table. 'I want you out of here soon,' she says 'as I need to move the furniture while I vacuum.   So why don't you go and have a nice bath and get dressed, the others will be getting up soon.'
I walk by the bathroom door but I don't enter instead I go back to my room where I quickly dress.
The day passes and my need for a cigarette becomes desperate, so much so that I return to the smoke room and light one up. I sit back feeling the pleasant rush of nicotine.   I get about half way through the cigarette when the voices remind me of my wickedness.
You're going to hell.
There's terrible things happening in the world and you're to blame.
I quickly crunch my cigarette out in the ash tray and burst into tears.

Then feeling like I've lost my only friend I throw the rest of the packet into the wastepaper basket and once again leave the smoke-room.

******

It's visiting time I watch out of the window as Pete gets out of his car.

He greets me with a peck on my forehead. 'How you feeling today?' he asks.

'She's all at sixes and sevens she's done nothing but pace the corridor all morning' says a woman who is standing by the door.

'Have you been having a bad day love?' asks Pete.

I shrug my shoulders.

'Come on we'll go to the office and I'll ask if I can take you out for a couple of hours a change of scenery might do you good.' I follow Pete as he walks up the corridor towards the office.

A nurse sits behind the desk, she happily grants Pete's request and together we leave the unit and walk towards Pete's car.

Once in the car Pete hands me a cigarette.

'I can't have one,' I mutter in a small voice.

'Don't try and stop smoking right now love I don't think it's the right time.'

'The voices won't let me.' I say.

'But I've told you before love, the voices aren't real.'

'Aren't they?'

'No so you sit back relax and have a smoke, try and ignore those damn voices.'

I take the cigarette and quickly light it. The voices don't return and for the first time that day I'm able to have a smoke in peace.

'Bloody hell it looks like there's been an accident.' Pete points to a police car and ambulance parked at the side of the road. I look out of the car window. Someone is lying on a stretcher and a man is been led inside the waiting ambulance.

You was the cause of that, screech the voices.

We warned you not to smoke.

As Pete drives away from the scene I burst into tears.

'What's wrong love.'

'It was all my fault I'm bad,' I mutter in between sobs,

'Don't cry love,' says Pete as he turns around and drives the car back towards Rosedale, 'you're not bad, you're just really, really ill.'

We   arrive back at on the unit to be greeted by a nurse,   ' Oh Lorraine I'm glad you're back,' she says , 'the doctor is doing her ward round early today,' 'and she's waiting to have a little chat with you.'

I say goodbye to Pete and follow the nurse into the doctor's clinic.

The doctor smiles at me, and looks me up and down.

'You look much better,' she says as she writes something down on the file in front of her.

I lower my head trying desperately to turn off my thoughts.

'I understand you have a holiday booked for next week, so I'm going to discharge you, just go home and have your holiday and you will be fine.' The doctor closes the file and I leave the clinic.

Chapter 30

'She's nowhere near to being discharged, 'says Pete later on that afternoon.

'That's the doctor's decision and this is only meant to be a short stay unit.' says the nurse.

'But she's only been in here a week and you don't have to be a doctor to see how ill she is.' Pete looks at me and sighs.

The nurse smiles 'well she can come back for day-care if she wants,' she says.

The nurse hands him my tablets 'perhaps that holiday will do you both the world of good,' she says.

'I'd almost forgotten about the holiday all I'm worried about is my wife I just want her well.' Says Pete as we leave the unit.

We arrive home Cheryl makes me a cup of tea, she seems glad to see me.

'Do you feel well enough to go to Spain, I mean we can always cancel it although it's a bit late in the day to get a refund,' says Pete.

Cheryl's looks on disappointed for she had looked so forward to going.,

I nod my head in fake enthusiasm, 'I'll be all-right, I say. 'Maybe the nurse was right, perhaps a holiday will help.'

******

I lie in the dark for hours unable to sleep so I go downstairs, automatically I light a cigarette. The voices all start talking at once. A lump forms in my throat, ashamed of myself I drop the cigarette in the ashtray praying nothing else bad will happen because of my thoughtlessness

The voice fade to a dull chant and it's impossible to make out what they are saying.

Presently I hear Pete coming down the stairs, 'can't you sleep love,' he says as he walks through the door I shake my head.

'Is it those voices? I wish I could take them away from you love,' he says as he sits by my side on the sofa, I'd do anything to get you well. I look at Pete and notice that his eyes are wet with unshed tears. At that moment I realise that I can trust him.

Pete places his arm protectively around my shoulders, there is little need for words as we sit in the semi darkness waiting for the day to begin.

******

Later on that morning Pete takes me back to Rosedale to begin my day-care.
A nurse meets us at the door, 'can you come back and pick your wife up at about eleven o'clock,' she asks.
'Eleven o' clock,' says Pete perplexed. 'I though Lorraine was having day care.
'She's only supposed to be here for two hours,' says the nurse.
Pete glances at the clock on the wall it reads ten fifteen, 'well there's hardly any point in her staying is there.' Pete takes my hand, 'come on love,' he says 'I'm taking you back home.'

Two days later I still haven't slept all sorts of thoughts are rushing inside my head. Sammy visits and takes me back to Rosedale where she begs the doctor to readmit me.
The doctor refuses muttering something about a shortage of beds and that I'm not a priority case.

******

It's the night before the holiday I try to force a smile on my face as Pete helps me pack my case. At seven thirty in morning we're catching the bus that will take us all the way to Spain Cheryl is very excited as she checks her passport for the tenth time that day.
Pete gives me a hug, 'get yourself to bed love,' he says as he zips up my case, 'we have a long day tomorrow.

It's getting light now, I've been awake for most of the night, the sleep I've had has been peppered with bad dreams. One of the dreams I had warned me of the peril we are in and what awaits us when we get to Spain. In the dream we were been stoned by the Spaniards as we ran across the beach the dream was so vivid.

The shrilling of the alarm clock wakes up Pete. He rubs the sleep from his eyes as he sits up in bed. 'We best get up love,' he says looking at the clock and giving me a gentle nudge, 'taxi will be here in an hour.

The cases are stood waiting in the hallway, Pete hears me sigh 'What's wrong love 'don't you want to go?'

I look up and see the disappointed look in Pete's eyes.
'If you don't feel well enough we don't have to go,' he says slowly.
'I'm okay,' I mutter.
However I'm afraid and find it difficult to dismiss the dream I had last night.
Suddenly Cheryl comes bounding down the stairs, ' Spain here we come she squeals at the top of her voice.

Before we know it the taxi arrives to take us to the pickup -point in the centre of Hull.
As we reach the gate I turn and take one last look at my house and then climb into the waiting taxi.
The bus is waiting for us at the pickup- point . Other passengers turn and glare at us as we board the bus,. The courier checks our tickets and shows us our seats.
'Do you want to sit near the window love?' asks Pete.
I shake my head and sit by his side and Cheryl sits just behind us.
The bus starts up and we're on our way. Very soon we have left Hull behind.
After some time we stop at a service station.
'Time to stretch your legs,' says the courier standing at the front of the bus.
I get up from my seat and make my way to the bus entrance Pete and Cheryl follow me.
The first thing Pete does when we get off the bus is to reach in his pocket for his cigarettes, he hands one to me. 'You might as well have a smoke,' he says, 'it'll be a long time before you can have another one.'
I hesitate and then take the cigarette which I light quickly. To my relief I am able to smoke it in peace.
After going to the toilet we get back on the bus.
'Are you sure you don't want to sit by the window?' asks Pete.
'Okay,' I say more to please him then myself.
The bus fills up with people and once again the driver starts up the engine.

You're bad.
We told you not to smoke.
Do you think we went away.
We know what you did.
I feel my body going rigid as I sit bolt upright in my seat.

Pete turns to me, 'are you feeling a bit nervous' he asks. 'Try to relax love have a little sleep you'll be alright when we get there just close your eyes and keep thinking of blue skies and golden sandy beaches.'

I close my eyes tightly but I can't shut out the dull rabble of the voices who are now having a conversation with each other inside my head.

She's a fool.
Yes she's an idiot and everyone despises her.
The voices gradually fade away, I sink back in my seat praying that they don't return. My head aches and my stomach feels numb. The hours pass by Pete tries to involve me in conversation but I ignore him as I know people are listening.

******

'We're at the docks,' says Cheryl excitedly, 'we'll be boarding the ferry soon.'

I glance out of the window and can see white cliffs looming against the grey sky.

Chapter 31

After two hours on the ferry we arrive in Calais.

With legs like jelly I board the bus which will take us from France to Spain.

I feel my stomach lurch as I sit back down in my seat a lady opposite me smiles. But I look away quickly because I know she is trying to read my mind.

The bus chugs on for hours, I stay silent, Pete sits doing a cross word puzzle after giving up all attempts to engage me in conversation.

The voices in my head are quite prominent now, they tell me that only Pete and Cheryl will be dropped off in Spain and I will have to stay on the bus where I will be taken to a place where I will be punished. I am so afraid my mouth feels dry like sandpaper and cold sweat runs down my back.

It's becoming very hot and uncomfortable on the bus and the further we travel the warmer it gets.

Eventually after an horrendously long and fearful journey we reach the Costa Bravo.

The bus stops outside a hotel.

'We're here,' says Cheryl, 'oh look at that swimming pool.'

We are shunted to the front of the bus and to my great relief the bus doors do not close in my face allowing me to step out to fresh air and clear blue skies.

Pete and Cheryl take the cases and looking carefully from left to right I follow them into the hotel where we are booked in and taken to the fourth floor to our rooms.

The room is large and airy we unpack our cases and Pete takes out our small travelling kettle, coffee and dried milk and sugar.

'I can't wait for a decent cup of coffee,' he says as he fills the kettle and plugs it in.

'That coffee we bought on the coach tasted like mud.'

The kettle soon boils Pete adds coffee to the cups and pours in the water he then hands me my cup. 'Now relax love,' he says 'you're on holiday now so try and forget your troubles and enjoy it. Have a smoke and chill out for a while before we shower and go and find somewhere nice to eat.'

Pete lights my cigarette and hands it me.

The voices erupt into a frenzy the moment I take a drag.
You wicked woman,
You've done it now,
You didn't pay heed to our warning.
I quickly lay the cigarette back in the ashtray.
Pete looks on and sighs. I feel his eyes looking into mine. 'You look a bit overwrought he says you might feel better after a shower, a change of clothes and some food inside you. I slowly undress and step into the shower the water splashes down on to my naked skin mingling with the tears that fall down my face.

******

'Aren't you going to eat something you must be starving you've hardly eaten in two days.'
I play about with the food on my plate ignoring my aching hunger pangs.
'Come on love just have a little bit.'
I shake my head and leave the table I walk out of the restaurant and sit at a table outside. People saunter by smiling couples hand in hand, laughing sun kissed children, everyone smiling everyone happy and carefree. Presently a man passes he has a long beard and his dark hair is reaching his waist. He gives me a knowing look as he passes and nods his head. I'm certain that he's Jesus.
Pete and Cheryl leave the restaurant, 'there was no need to have just walked out,' says Pete a little annoyed, 'you could have waited while me and Cheryl had finished our meal even if you didn't want to eat.'
'Come on lets go on the beach,' says Cheryl eager to change the subject.
Reluctantly I follow Pete and Cheryl to the sea front, I'm so afraid, there are people everywhere and they are all discussing my downfall. The beach is packed we hire our sun-beds and Pete and Cheryl lie back I sit on the edge of mine keeping my head down.
'For Gods sake will you just chill out,' says Pete.
I ignore him and stay where I am at the edge of the sun-bed and cover my face with my hands.
After about an hour Pete gives up trying to coax me and we slowly make our way back to our hotel.

'I should never have brought you here,' says Pete, I knew you wasn't well you should still be in hospital I tried to tell that doctor but she just wouldn't listen to me.

'I'm going to lie by the pool,' says Cheryl she shrugs her shoulders and leaves the room.

Come on we'll go and sit on the balcony.'

Reluctantly I follow Pete out on to the balcony, we sit on plastic chairs at a small table once again Pete takes out his crossword book. Our balcony overlooks a small tiled patio I look down a man is sweeping the floor he waves at us and smiles.

That man is your enemy.

Don't be deceived by him. He hates you really.

The voices echo around my head, trembling I go back inside the hotel room.

I sit huddled in a chair me eyes darting from left to right looking for a webcam that has been hidden to record my every movement.

Chapter 32

It's the fourth day of our holiday and I'm terrified I have hardly slept or eaten since I came here. The voices have plagued me for most of the day. They tell me that something terrible is going to happen to my family Pete is very worried about me and tries in vain to convince me that the voices aren't real but I don't believe him for they are so vivid and clear.

I pace up and down the floor of the hotel room Pete is in the shower and the voices are screeching and screaming out their threats.
They're coming tonight.
They're going to take you to a place where you will never be free.
My mind in a turmoil I continue pacing up and down up and down.
They're going to get you all.
In the dead of the night they will put Pete against a wall and shoot him.
My heart beats wildly I'm so afraid I can feel my hair prickle the back of my neck.
You're wicked,
Older than time,
You deserve to suffer for your sins.
They're coming very soon.
Unable to bear it any longer I dash out on to the balcony standing on the plastic chair I climb backwards over the edge. I cling on to the railings then quickly I release my grip.

Where am I? the pavement is sloping the pain is intense I look up towards the large building it then comes back to me the hotel, the balcony, the voices. Pete is looking down at me from the balcony 'Lorraine Lorraine,' he screams 'oh why.
I try to sit up I cry out in pain and am forced to stay laid down.

A siren rings in my ears I feel myself been lifted up and carried away on some sort of stretcher.
Someone is stroking my hair 'try not to move,' says a voice' in broken English 'that's it keep still we are taking you to the hospital.
I close my eyes against the pain and fade away into the blackness.

I'm lying on a board in a large white room, I want to cry out but the pain is taking my breath away. I see a face hovering over me.
'Please take me off this board,' I say in between gasps, 'it hurts so much.'
'You are not lying on a board you are on a bed. You have broken your back, I have just seen your x-ray results. And your pelvis and ankles, they are also broken.'
I want Pete,' I cry, 'where's Pete, is he alright?' I look up the face has disappeared.
I lie there for what seems like hours I close my eyes tightly against the pain and the fear. Questions run around and round in my head *am I dying will I ever see my girls again. Pete where are you, where are you.*

******

The police translator sits by my bed by her side is a man who I have not seen before.
'Do you remember what happened Mrs Ellis,' says the translater.
'Where's Pete?'
'He's with the police we need to get to the bottom of what happened on the balcony,'
The man says something in Spanish to the courier who then turns to me.'
'How did you fall off the balcony?' she asks where you pushed?'
I shake my head.
'Is your husband a violent man does ever he hit you?'
'No never.'
I moan overcome by a wave of pain.
The translator looks on Sympathetically, 'I'll try and get them to give you some morphine,' she says.
I climbed off the balcony held on to the railings and then let go,' I say slowly.
'So you tried to commit sucide?'
'No I was frightened I needed to escape.'
'Escape?'
'Escape from the voices in my head, they told me there were going to hurt my family kill Pete_'
The translator looks at me long and hard, 'do you hear voices,' she asks.

I nod my head, tears of physical and mental anguish fall down my cheeks. 'I want Pete' I cry 'is he alright?'

The translator's face softens, 'Your husband's fine you'll see him soon.' Everything will be sorted out now, no one is going to hurt anyone you are quite safe.' She turns to the man and speaks to him in Spanish she then turns to me and pats my arm, 'I should think your husband will be here soon,' she says before her and the man both leave my bedside.'

And so the hours pass, hours of pain, hours of fear where I drift in and out of consciousness.

Am I dreaming I can hear him call my name softly and slowly I can feel a hand stroking my forehead.

I open my eyes and to my utter relief Pete is standing by my bed, Cheryl stands by his side.

'Oh Lorraine love I've been so worried about you.' .

I want to sit up and throw my arms around Pete, make sure I'm not dreaming but the pain won't let me.

He's still alive he hasn't been killed the voices they have tricked me.

'Try and keep still mam,' says Cheryl,

'Oh why did you do it love,' says Pete.

'I was scared,' I mutter, 'so scared.'

Pete sighs sadly, 'I wouldn't let anyone ever hurt you,' he says.

I look up into Pete's eyes and I begin to feel safe.

'Was it the voices again?' says Pete.

'Yes there were saying some terrible things.'

'Have they gone now.'

'I can't hear then anymore.'

'Good, just keep telling yourself that there were part of the illness you must believe that.'

'I'll try,' I mutter, 'but there were so real.

'It was all a bad dream,' says Pete gently and dreams aren't real are they.'

Chapter 33

I have been in the Spanish hospital for a week now and it has been decided that I will be better off having the operation on my left ankle done in England. So today I will be airlifted back to England and taken to Hull Royal infirmary. There will only be room for a nurse and another person to accompany me back in the plane to England. So It has been arranged for Pete to travel home with the holiday firm and for Cheryl to come home with me on the aeroplane. I have been given some morphine which to my relief has taken the edge off the pain.

My transport soon arrives to take me to the airport, the rest of the time passes in a haze and the next thing I know is that I'm lying on a stretcher in the aeroplane. Cheryl and the nurse sit by my side. No one speaks much on the journey home Cheryl looks at me her face etched with worry and I'm consumed with guilt. Thoughts spin around in my head, *why did I listen to the voice, they wasn't real there was no one there, you should have known better, it's happened before you should have known better.*

It's late afternoon when we arrive back in England where I'm taken to Hull Royal infirmary. The morphine is beginning to wear off and I feel sick with pain.

I'm admitted to the hospital and taken to a ward where a nurse does her best to make me feel comfortable. Cheryl sits by my bed, she looks tired so I insist that she goes home and rests.

The pain comes in white hot waves I try to remember the breathing I'd learnt during the birth of my babies and this helps a little. However this is very difficult as the pain seems to be taking over my whole body. A nurse attaches me to a drip and after a while the pain eases slightly.

Later on I'm taken for another x-ray, I feel every movement as the nurses carefully eases me on to a trolley. The porter then takes me down in the lift, he seems a cheerful man but I fear him as I feel he's come to check up on me. I then reproach myself for my strange thought which I'm slowly beginning to believe is paranoia a part of my illness.

The next morning the hospital physiatrist arrives to talk to me she seems a nice lady and although I have never seen her before I feel that I can trust her, She decides to change my medication and puts me on a drug called olanzapine.

******

A group of doctors stand around my bed, the consultant looks in my notes.

'How are you feeling today?' he asks.

'Will I ever walk again?' I ask ignoring his question.

'We need to operate on your ankle soon but we feel that after three months bed rest your back will have grown new bone-'

'But will I walk again?'

'I hope so,' says the consultant. After giving me a reassuring smile he leaves my bedside along with the group of doctors.

******

After my operation I wake up in the high dependency unit where I stay for four days under the dedicated care of the staff.

I have had bone taken from my hip and grafted into my ankle along with pins and a plate to hold my bones together.

The doctor tells me that my operation has been a success and in time I will walk again.

However he says my ankle and back will always be weak and I will always have a limp.

Epilogue

I stayed in hospital for twelve weeks having had eleven weeks bed rest.

I strongly believe that it was this complete rest, the dedication of the staff and perhaps a change in medication that helped me to recover my mental health.

After eleven weeks I made my first stumbling steps it was extremely painful made more difficult by the cumbersome back brace I had to wear. Much to my relief the brace was taken off six weeks later.

Today my walking has improved, however I have to use a wheel chair for long distances. I still get a lot of pain in my ankle. And I suffer a lot with backache as my back didn't set properly and my spine is now slightly curved.

Samantha was blessed with a beautiful daughter who was quickly followed by two more.

Pete and Cheryl and I moved into a bungalow in the small village of Paull it was to be a fresh start for us.

Much to my delight Lucy and the family were reunited she now has a lovely little girl.

Fortunately I haven't had a breakdown in my mental health for seven years now and I have recently been discharged from the mental health services Although I need to take medication for the rest of my life, but I feel that it's a small price to pay for my sanity.

I have taken up writing again and have finished writing my novel: Pease Pudding Hot. Which to my delight has been accepted for publication by chipmunkapublishing.com a mental health publishers whose aim is to give a voice to people affected by mental illness.

I smile to myself as I stand at the window watching my grandchildren at play and I feel overcome with happiness.

Lightning Source UK Ltd.
Milton Keynes UK
03 April 2011

170314UK00001B/10/P